BRADY

PARAMEDIC CARE: PRINCIPLES & PRACTICE

TRAUMA EMERGENCIES

Workbook

Robert S. Porter

BRYAN E. BLEDSOE, D.O., F.A.C.E.P., F.A.A.E.M., F.A.E.P., EMT-P
Emergency Department Staff Physician
Baylor Medical Center—Ellis County
Waxahachie, Texas
and
Clinical Associate Professor of Emergency Medicine
University of North Texas Health Sciences Center
Fort Worth, Texas

ROBERT S. PORTER, M.A., NREMT-P
Senior Advanced Life Support Educator
Madison County Emergency Medical Services
Canastota, New York
and
Flight Paramedic
AirOne, Onondaga County Sheriff's Department
Syracuse, New York

RICHARD A. CHERRY, M.S., NREMT-P
Clinical Assistant Professor of Emergency Medicine
Director of Paramedic Training
SUNY Upstate Medical University
Syracuse, New York

Prentice Hall

Upper Saddle River, New Jersey 07458

Dedication

*To Kris and sailing: Pleasant distractions from writing about
and practicing prehospital emergency medicine.*

PUBLISHER: *Julie Alexander*
EXECUTIVE EDITOR: *Greg Vis*
MANAGING DEVELOPMENT EDITOR: *Lois Berlowitz*
DEVELOPMENT EDITOR: *Dan Zinkus*
MARKETING MANAGER: *Tiffany Price*
DIRECTOR OF MANUFACTURING & PRODUCTION:
  Bruce Johnson
SENIOR PRODUCTION MANAGER: *Ilene Sanford*
MANAGING PRODUCTION EDITOR: *Patrick Walsh*
PRODUCTION SUPERVISION: *Navta Associates, Inc.*
PRINTER/BINDER: *Banta Harrisonburg*

© 2001 by Pearson Education, Inc.
Upper Saddle River, New Jersey 07458

Printed in the United States of America
10 9 8 7 6 5 4 3

ISBN 0-13-021641-0

Prentice-Hall International (UK) Limited, *London*
Prentice-Hall of Australia Pty. Limited, *Sydney*
Prentice-Hall Canada Inc., *Toronto*
Prentice-Hall Hispanoamericana, S.A., *Mexico*
Prentice-Hall of India Private Limited, *New Delhi*
Prentice-Hall of Japan, Inc., *Tokyo*
Prentice-Hall (Singapore) Pte Ltd
Editora Prentice-Hall do Brasil, Ltda., *Rio de Janeiro*

NOTICE ON CARE PROCEDURES

It is the intent of the authors and publisher that this
workbook be used as part of a formal EMT-Paramedic
program taught by qualified instructors and supervised
by a licensed physician. The procedures described in
this workbook are based upon consultation with EMT
and medical authorities. The authors and publisher
have taken care to make certain that these procedures
reflect currently accepted clinical practice; however,
they cannot be considered absolute recommendations.

The material in this workbook contains the most
current information available at the time of publica-
tion. However, federal, state, and local guidelines con-
cerning clinical practices, including, without limitation,
those governing infection control and universal precautions, change rapidly. The reader should note, there-
fore, that the new regulations may require changes in
some procedures.

It is the responsibility of the reader to familiarize
himself or herself with the policies and procedures set
by federal, state, and local agencies as well as the institution or agency where the reader is employed. The
authors and the publisher of this workbook disclaim
any liability, loss, or risk resulting directly or indirectly
from the suggested procedures and theory, from any
undetected errors, or from the reader's misunderstand-
ing of the text. It is the reader's responsibility to stay
informed of any new changes or recommendations
made by any federal, state, and local agency as well as
by his or her employing institution or agency.

CONTENTS

Self-Instructional Workbook

Paramedic Care: Principles & Practice

TRAUMA EMERGENCIES

INTRODUCTION
To the Self-Instructional Workbook
Paramedic Care: Principles & Practice

Welcome to the self-instructional workbook for *Paramedic Care: Principles & Practice*. This workbook is designed to help guide you through an educational program for initial or refresher training that follows the guidelines of the 1998 U.S. Department of Transportation EMT-Paramedic National Standard Curriculum. The workbook is designed to be used either in conjunction with your instructor or as a self-study guide you use on your own.

This workbook features many different ways to help you learn the material necessary to become a paramedic, including those listed below.

FEATURES

Review of Chapter Objectives
Each chapter of *Paramedic Care: Principles & Practice* begins with objectives that identify the important information and principles addressed in the chapter reading. To help you identify and learn this material, each workbook chapter reviews the important content elements addressed by these objectives as presented in the text.

Case Study Review
Each chapter of *Paramedic Care: Principles & Practice* includes a case study, introducing and highlighting important principles presented in the chapter. The workbook reviews these case studies and points out much of the essential information and many of the applied principles they describe.

Content Self-Evaluation
Each chapter of *Paramedic Care: Principles & Practice* presents an extensive narrative explanation of the principles of paramedic practice. The workbook chapter (or chapter section) contains between 10 and 90 multiple-choice questions to test your reading comprehension of the textbook material and to give you experience taking typical emergency medical service examinations.

Special Projects
The workbook contains several projects that are special learning experiences designed to help you remember the information and principles necessary to perform as a paramedic. Special projects include crossword puzzles, personal benchmarking activities, and a variety of other exercises.

Personal Benchmarking
The workbook provides exercises that ask you to practice using your body and your observations of the world around you to develop and refine your skills of assessing patients and analyzing scenes to which you are called for mechanisms of injury.

Chapter Sections
Several chapters in *Paramedic Care: Principles & Practice* are long and contain a great deal of subject matter. To help you grasp this material more efficiently, the workbook breaks these chapters into sections with their own objectives, content review, and special projects.

Content Review
The workbook provides a comprehensive review of the material presented in this volume of *Paramedic Care: Principles & Practice*. After the last text chapter has been covered, the workbook presents an

extensive content self-evaluation component that helps you recall and build upon the knowledge you have gained by reading the text, attending class, and completing the earlier workbook chapters.

National Registry Practical Evaluation Forms

Supplemental materials found at the back of the workbook include the National Registry Practical Evaluation Forms. These or similar forms will be used to test your practical skills throughout your training and, usually, for state certification exams. By reviewing them, you have a clearer picture of what is expected of you during your practical exam and a better understanding of the type of evaluation tool that is used to measure your performance.

Patient Scenario Flash Cards

This workbook contains 3″ × 5″ cards, each of which presents a patient scenario with signs and symptoms. On the reverse side is the appropriate field diagnosis and the care steps you should consider providing for the patient. These cards will help you recognize and remember common serious trauma emergencies, their presentation, and the appropriate care that should be given.

ACKNOWLEDGMENTS

Reviewers
The reviewers listed below provided many excellent suggestions for improving this workbook. Their assistance is greatly appreciated.

Edward B. Kuvlesky, NREMT-P
Battalion Chief
Indian River County EMS
Indian River County, Florida

K. Lee Watson, NREMT-P
Martinsville-Henry County Rescue Squad
Martinsville, Virginia

How to Use

The Self-Instructional Workbook

Paramedic Care: Principles & Practice

The self-instructional workbook accompanying *Paramedic Care: Principles & Practice* may be used as directed by your instructor or independently by you during your course of instruction. The recommendations listed below are intended to guide you in using the workbook independently.

- Examine your course schedule and identify the appropriate text chapter or other assigned reading.

- Read the assigned chapter in *Paramedic Care: Principles & Practice* carefully. Do this in a relaxed environment, free of distractions, and give yourself adequate time to read and digest the material. The information presented in *Paramedic Care: Principles & Practice* is often technically complex and demanding, but it is very important that you comprehend it. Be sure that you read the chapter carefully enough to understand and remember what you have read.

- Carefully read the Review of Chapter Objectives at the beginning of each workbook chapter (or section). This material includes both the objectives listed in *Paramedic Care: Principles & Practice* and narrative descriptions of their content. If you do not understand or remember what is discussed from your reading, refer to the referenced pages and reread them carefully. If you still do not feel comfortable with your understanding of any objective, consider asking your instructor about it.

- Reread the case study in *Paramedic Care: Principles & Practice,* and then read the Case Study Review in the workbook. Note the important points regarding assessment and care that the Case Study Review highlights and be sure that you understand and agree with the analysis of the call. If you have any questions or concerns, ask your instructor to clarify the information.

- Take the Content Self-Evaluation at the end of each workbook chapter (or section), answering each question carefully. Do this in a quiet environment, free from distractions, and allow yourself adequate time to complete the exercise. Correct your self-evaluation by consulting the answers at the back of the workbook, and determine the percentage you have answered correctly (the number you got right divided by the total number of questions). If you have answered most of the questions correctly (85 to 90 percent), review those that you missed by rereading the material on the pages listed in the answer key and be sure you understand which answer is correct and why. If you have more than a few questions wrong (less than 85 percent correct), look for incorrect answers that are grouped together. This suggests that you did not understand a particular topic in the reading. Reread the text dealing with that topic carefully, and then retest yourself on the questions you got wrong. If incorrect answers are spread throughout the chapter content, reread the chapter and retake the Content Self-Evaluation to assure that you understand the material. If you don't understand why your answer to a question is incorrect after reviewing the text, consult with your instructor.

- In a similar fashion, complete the exercises in the Special Projects section of the workbook chapters (or sections). These exercises are specifically designed to help you learn and remember the essential principles and information presented in *Paramedic Care: Principles & Practice.*

- When you have completed this volume of *Paramedic Care: Principles & Practice* and its accompanying workbook, prepare for a course test by reviewing both the text in its entirety and your class notes. Then take the Content Review examination in the workbook. Again, review your score and any questions you have answered incorrectly by referring to the text and rereading the page or pages where the material is presented. If you note groupings of wrong answers, review the entire range of pages or the full chapter they represent.

If, during your completion of the workbook exercises, you have any questions that either the textbook or workbook doesn't answer, write them down and ask your instructor about them. Prehospital emergency medicine is a complex and complicated subject, and answers are not always black-and-white. It is also common for different EMS systems to use differing methods of care. The questions you bring up in class, and your instructor's answers to them, will help you expand and complete your knowledge of prehospital emergency medical care.

The authors and Brady Publishing continuously seek to ensure the creation of the best materials to support your educational experience. We are interested in your comments. If, during your reading and study of material in *Paramedic Care: Principles & Practice*, you notice any error or have any suggestions to improve either the textbook or workbook, please use the comment form at the back of this workbook. Alternatively, you can direct your comments via the Internet to the following address:

harrier@localnet.com

You can also visit the Brady website at:
www.bradybooks.com/paramedic

GUIDELINES TO BETTER TEST-TAKING

The knowledge you will gain from reading the textbook, completing the exercises in the workbook, listening in your paramedic class, and participating in your clinical and field experience will prepare you to care for patients who are seriously ill or injured. However, before you can practice these skills, you will have to pass several classroom written exams and your state's certification exam successfully. Your performance on these exams will depend not only on your knowledge but also on your ability to answer test questions correctly. The following guidelines are designed to help your performance on tests and to better demonstrate your knowledge of prehospital emergency care.

1. Relax and be calm during the test.

A test is designed to measure what you have learned and to tell you and your instructor how well you are doing. An exam is not designed to intimidate or punish you. Consider it a challenge, and just try to do your best. Get plenty of sleep prior to the examination. Avoid coffee or other stimulants for a few hours before the exam, and be prepared.

Reread the text chapters, review the objectives in the workbook, and review your class notes. It might be helpful to work with one or two other students and ask each other questions. This type of practice helps everyone better understand the knowledge presented in your course of study.

2. Read the questions carefully.

Read each word of the question and all the answers slowly. Words such as "except" or "not" may change the entire meaning of the question. If you miss such words, you may answer the question incorrectly even though you know the right answer.

EXAMPLE:
The art and science of Emergency Medical Services involves all of the following EXCEPT:

    A. sincerity and compassion.
    B. respect for human dignity.
    C. placing patient care before personal safety.
    D. delivery of sophisticated emergency medical care.
    E. none of the above

The correct answer is C, unless you miss the "EXCEPT."

3. Read each answer carefully.

Read each and every answer carefully. While the first answer may be absolutely correct, so may the rest, and thus the best answer might be "all of the above."

EXAMPLE:
Indirect medical control is considered to be:

    A. treatment protocols.
    B. training and education.
    C. quality assurance.
    D. chart review.
    E. all of the above

While answers A, B, C, and D are correct, the best and only acceptable answer is "all of the above," E.

4. Delay answering questions you don't understand and look for clues.

When a question seems confusing or you don't know the answer, note it on your answer sheet and come back to it later. This will ensure that you have time to complete the test. You will also find that other questions in the test may give you hints to answer the one you've skipped over. It will also prevent you from being frustrated with an early question and letting it affect your performance.

EXAMPLE:
Upon successful completion of a course of training as an EMT-P, most states will

    A. certify you. (correct)
    B. license you.
    C. register you.
    D. recognize you as a paramedic.
    E. issue you a permit.

Another question, later in the exam, may suggest the right answer:

The action of one state in recognizing the certification of another is called:

    A. reciprocity. (correct)
    B. national registration.
    C. licensure.
    D. registration.
    E. extended practice.

5. Answer all questions.

Even if you do not know the right answer, do not leave a question blank. A blank question is always wrong, while a guess might be correct. If you can eliminate some of the answers as wrong, do so. It will increase the chances of a correct guess.

EXAMPLE:
When a paramedic is called by the patient (through the dispatcher) to the scene of a medical emergency, the medical control physician has established a physician/patient relationship.

    A. True
    B. False

    A true/false question gives you a 50 percent chance of a correct guess.

The hospital health professional responsible for sorting patients as they arrive at the emergency department is usually the:

    A. emergency physician.
    B. ward clerk.
    C. emergency nurse.
    D. trauma surgeon.
    E. both A and C (correct)

    A multiple-choice question with five answers gives a 20 percent chance of a correct guess. If you can eliminate one or more incorrect answers, you increase your odds of a correct guess to 25 percent, 33 percent, and so on. An unanswered question has a 0 percent chance of being correct.
    Just before turning in your answer sheet, check to be sure that you have not left any items blank.

CHAPTER 1
*
Trauma and Trauma Systems

Review of Chapter Objectives

After reading this chapter, you should be able to:

1. Describe the prevalence and significance of trauma. pp. 5–6

Trauma is the fourth most common cause of mortality and the number one killer for persons under the age of 44. It accounts for about 150,000 deaths per year and may be the most expensive medical problem of society today. Traumas can be divided into those caused by blunt and penetrating injury mechanisms, with only 10 percent of all trauma patients experiencing life-threatening injuries and the need for the services of the trauma center/system.

2. List the components of a comprehensive trauma system. pp. 6–8

The trauma system consists of a state-level agency that coordinates regional trauma systems. The regional systems consist of regional, area, and community trauma centers and, in some cases, other facilities designated and dedicated to the care of trauma patients. The trauma system also consists of injury prevention, provider education, data registry, and quality assurance programs.

3. Identify the characteristics of community, area, and regional trauma centers. p. 7

Community or Level III Trauma Center. This is a general hospital with a commitment to provide resources and staff training specific to the care of trauma patients. Such centers are generally located in rural areas and will stabilize the more serious trauma patients, and then transport them to higher level trauma centers.

Area or Level II Trauma Center. This is a facility with an increased commitment to trauma patient care including 24-hour surgery. A Level II center can handle all but the most critical and specialty trauma patients.

Regional or Level I Trauma Center. This is a facility, usually a university teaching hospital, that is staffed and equipped to handle all types of serious trauma 24 hours a day and 7 days a week, as well as to support and oversee the regional trauma system.

In some areas there is a Level IV trauma facility, which receives trauma patients and stabilizes them for transport to a higher level facility.

4. Identify the trauma triage criteria and apply them to several narrative descriptions of trauma patients. pp. 9–12

Trauma triage criteria include a listing of mechanisms of injury and physical findings suggestive of serious injury. The criteria identify patients likely to benefit from the care offered by the Level I or II trauma center. They include:

Mechanism of Injury

Falls greater than 20 feet (3x victim's height)
Motorcycle accidents (over 20 mph)
Severe vehicle impacts
Death of another vehicle occupant

Pedestrian/bicyclist vs. auto collisions
Ejections from vehicles
Rollovers with serious impact
Prolonged extrications

Physical Findings

Revised Trauma Score less than 11
Glasgow Coma Scale less than 14
Pulse greater than 120 or less than 50
Multiple proximal long bone fractures
Pelvic fractures
Respiratory rate greater than 29 or less than 10
Burns greater than 15% body surface area (BSA)

Pediatric Trauma Score less than 9
Systolic blood pressure less than 90
Penetrating trauma (non-extremity)
Flail chest
Limb paralysis
Airway or facial burns

5. Describe how trauma differs from medical emergencies in the scene size-up, assessment, prehospital emergency care, and transport. pp. 9–12

Scene size-up of the trauma incident differs from that with the medical emergency in that it is usually associated with more numerous scene hazards and involves an analysis of the mechanism of injury, using the evidence of impact to suggest possible injuries (the index of suspicion).

Assessment employs an initial assessment examining the risk of spinal injury, a quick mental status check, and an evaluation of airway, breathing, and circulation (ABCs), followed by a rapid trauma assessment looking to the head and torso and any sites of potential serious injury suggested by the index of suspicion or patient complaint.

Prehospital care and *transport* of the trauma patient is designed to provide expedient and supportive care and rapid transport of the patient to the trauma center or other appropriate facility.

6. Explain the "Golden Hour" concept and describe how it applies to prehospital emergency medical service. pp. 10–11

Research has demonstrated that the seriously injured trauma patient has an increasing chance for survival as the time from the injury to surgical intervention is reduced. Practically, this time should be as short as possible, ideally less than one hour. This "Golden Hour" concept directs prehospital care providers to reduce on-scene and transport times by expeditious assessment and care at the scene and by the use of air medical transport when appropriate and available.

7. Explain the value of air medical service in trauma patient care and transport. pp. 10–11

Air medical transport can move the trauma patient more quickly and along a direct line from the crash scene to the trauma center, thereby reducing transport time and increasing the likelihood that the patient will reach definitive care expeditiously.

CASE STUDY REVIEW

Reread the case study on pages 3 and 4 in Paramedic Care: Trauma Emergencies *before reading the discussion below.*

This case study presents a good opportunity to examine the components of the trauma system and the role they fulfill in the provision of prehospital care. John's very life is dependent upon the trauma system functioning efficiently.

Paramedic Earl Antak responds to the incident alone in a vehicle with advanced life support equipment, but not designed to transport patients (sometimes called a fly car). This system configuration permits advanced life support to be more flexible and available to a larger geographic area. Less seriously injured patients may be transported by ambulance without the paramedic, making John more quickly available for another call, or in this case available immediately after the helicopter leaves with the patient.

As Earl arrives at the scene he performs the elements of the scene survey. He assures the scene is safe and that the police are controlling traffic. Earl, in consideration of scene safety, will don gloves as there are open wounds, and he avoids the glass around the vehicle door. As he approaches the patient, Earl evaluates the mechanism of injury and notes that the bicyclist probably ran into the open car door. The mechanism of injury suggests significant impact and the probable need to enter the patient into the trauma system. Earl also notes that the rider was wearing a helmet, possibly the result of injury prevention programs in his local community, and suggesting a reduced incidence of head injuries, though not reducing the chances of spinal injury.

Earl's initial assessment reveals a well-developed young male who was unconscious but now is fully conscious and alert. Earl rules out any immediate airway, breathing, or circulation problem, applies oxygen, and ensures that the sheriff's department officer and then the ambulance crew continue to maintain immobilization of John's head and spine. As Earl moves on to the rapid trauma assessment, he notes neurologic signs that suggest a cervical spine injury. Earl also notes a likely clavicle fracture and carefully assesses for any associated respiratory injury. He also carefully watches for the early signs of shock, because clavicular injury can lacerate the subclavian artery. Vital signs are within normal limits for someone recently involved in heavy exercise and the emotional stress of trauma. Earl will, however, carefully record the vital signs and the results of his rapid trauma assessment during the ongoing assessments (every 5 minutes for this patient) and compare them to detect any trends in the patient's condition.

Earl contacts Medical Control and is assigned a transport destination. This communication ensures that John is transported to an appropriate center and one that has the resources to care for his injuries. Should a particular center be overcrowded with patients or have essential services unavailable (as, for example, no surgeon immediately on hand), Earl would be directed to transport John to another facility. As time is a critical factor in caring for John, Earl quickly performs the skills necessary to protect John's spine, then moves to transport him quickly. Earl also requests air medical services because the ground transport time is in excess of 30 minutes. He does not, however, await the helicopter but intercepts it at a predesignated landing zone. His intercept with the helicopter will likely reduce the transport time by minutes, an important factor with a seriously injured trauma patient. In this case, it is clearly to John's benefit to get to the trauma center as quickly as possible. The interactions between Earl and the police officer, the responding EMTs in the ambulance, the medical direction physician, the trauma triage nurse, and the flight crew ensure that the system works in a coordinated way and to the benefit of its patient, John.

CONTENT SELF-EVALUATION

MULTIPLE CHOICE

_____ 1. Auto accidents account for how many deaths each year?
   A. 12,000
   B. 24,000
   C. 44,000
   D. 68,000
   E. 150,000

_____ 2. Although trauma poses a serious threat to life, its presentation often masks the patient's true condition.
   A. True
   B. False

_____ 3. Some 90 percent of all trauma patients do not have serious, life-endangering injuries.
   A. True
   B. False

_____ 4. Trauma triage criteria are mechanisms of injury or physical signs exhibited by the patient that suggest serious injury.
   A. True
   B. False

_____ 5. The legislation that led to the development of today's Emergency Medical Services system was the:
   A. Trauma Care Systems Planning and Development Act of 1970.
   B. Consolidated Emergency Services Act of 1971.
   C. Highway Safety Act of 1966.
   D. Trauma Systems Act of 1963.
   E. National Readiness Act of 1960.

_____ 6. The trauma system is predicated on the principle that serious trauma is:
   A. a frequent occurrence.
   B. usually a medical emergency.
   C. inevitable.
   D. a surgical disease.
   E. fatal if the patient is not seen by a qualified physician in less than 30 minutes.

_____ 7. A Level I trauma center is usually a(n):
   A. community hospital.
   B. teaching hospital with resources available full-time for emergency cases.
   C. emergency department with 24-hour service.
   D. non-emergency health care facility.
   E. stabilizing and transport facility.

_____ 8. The small community hospital or healthcare facility in a remote area, designated as a receiving facility for trauma, is Level:
   A. I.   D. IV.
   B. II.   E. V.
   C. III.

_____ 9. Trauma centers may also be designated for provision of which of the following special services?
   A. pediatric trauma center   D. hyperbaric center
   B. burn center   E. all of the above
   C. neurocenter

_____ 10. The period of time between the occurrence of serious injury and surgery suggested as a goal for prehospital care providers is the:
   A. platinum 10 minutes.   D. bleed-out equation.
   B. golden hour.   E. critical differential.
   C. trauma time differential.

_____ 11. In applying trauma triage criteria, it is best to err on the side of precaution.
   A. True
   B. False

_____ 12. Trauma triage criteria are designed to over-triage trauma patients to ensure those with more subtle injuries are not missed.
   A. True
   B. False

_____ 13. The reduction in the incidence and seriousness of trauma in recent years can be credited to:
   A. better highway design.
   B. better auto design.
   C. use of auto restraint systems.
   D. development of injury prevention programs.
   E. all of the above

_____ 14. The standardized data retrieval system used to evaluate and improve the trauma system is the:
   A. prehospital care report system.   D. trauma quality improvement program.
   B. trauma triage system.   E. CISD.
   C. trauma registry.

_____ 15. Quality Improvement is a significant method of assessing system quality and providing for its improvement.
   A. True
   B. False

CHAPTER 2
Blunt Trauma

Review of Chapter Objectives

After reading this chapter, you should be able to:

1. Identify, and explain by example, the laws of inertia and conservation of energy.   pp. 20–21

Inertia is the tendency for objects at rest or in motion to remain so unless acted upon by an outside force. In some cases, that force is the energy exchange that causes trauma. For example, a bullet will continue its travel until it exchanges all its energy with the tissue it strikes.

Conservation of energy is the physical law explaining that energy is not lost but changes form in the auto or other impact. An example is the deformity in the auto when it impacts a tree.

2. Define kinetic energy and force as they relate to trauma.   pp. 20–23

Kinetic energy is the energy any moving object possesses. This energy is the potential to do harm if it is distributed to a victim.

Force is the exchange of energy from one object to another. It is determined by an object's mass (weight) and the velocity of rate change (acceleration or deceleration). This force induces injury.

3. Compare and contrast the types of vehicle impacts and their expected injuries.   pp. 23–26, 28–42

There are basically five types of vehicle impacts—frontal, lateral, rotational, rear-end, or rollover impacts. There are four events within each impact. First, the vehicle impacts the object and quickly comes to rest. Then, the vehicle occupant impacts the vehicle interior and comes to rest. Meanwhile, various organs and structures within the occupant's body collide with one another causing compression and stretching and injury. In the fourth event, objects within the vehicle may continue their forward motion until they impact the slowed or stopped occupant. In some instances, secondary vehicle impacts occur; these are impacts that may subject the injured occupant to additional acceleration, deceleration, and injury.

Frontal impact is the most common type of auto collision, although it also offers the most structural protection for the occupant. The front crumple zones of the auto absorb energy and the restraints—seat belts and airbags—provide additional protection. The anterior surface of the victim impacts the steering wheel, dash, windshield and/or firewall resulting in chest, abdominal, head, and neck injuries as well as knee, femur, and hip fractures.

Lateral impacts occur without the benefit of the front crumple zones, thereby permitting transmission of more energy directly to the occupant. The occupant is turned 90 degrees to the impact, resulting in fractures of the hip, femur, shoulder girdle, clavicle, and lateral ribs. Internal injury may result to the aorta and spleen on the driver's side or liver on the passenger's side. An unbelted occupant may impact the other occupant, causing further injury.

Rotational impacts result from oblique contact between vehicles, spinning as well as slowing the autos. This mediates the deceleration and reduces the expected injury. Injury patterns resemble a mix of those associated with frontal and lateral patterns though the severity is generally reduced.

Rear-end impacts push the auto, auto seat, and finally the occupant forward. The body is well protected, though the head may remain stationary while the shoulders move rapidly forward. The result may be hyperextension of the head and neck and cervical spine injury. Once the vehicle begins deceleration, other injuries may occur as the body contacts the dash, steering wheel, or windshield if the occupant is unbelted.

Rollovers occur as the roadway elevation changes or a vehicle with a high center of gravity becomes unstable around a turn. The vehicle impacts the ground as it turns, exposing the occupants to multiple impacts in places where the vehicle interior may be not designed to absorb such impacts. The result may be serious injuries to anywhere on the body or ejection of the occupants. Restraints greatly reduce the incidence of injury and ejection, while ejection greatly increases the chance of occupant death.

4. Discuss the benefits of auto restraint and motorcycle helmet use.   pp. 26–28, 39

Lap belts and shoulder straps control the deceleration of the vehicle occupant during a crash, slowing them with the auto. The result is a great reduction in injuries and deaths. However, when improperly worn, serious injuries may result. Shoulder straps alone may account for serious neck injury while the lap belt worn too high may injure the spine and abdomen.

Airbags inflate explosively during an impact and provide a cushion of gas as the occupant impacts the steering wheel, dash, or vehicle side. This slows the impact, reduces the deceleration rate, and reduces injuries. The airbag may entrap the driver's fingers and result in fractures or may impact a small driver or passenger who is seated close to the device and result in facial injury.

Child safety seats provide much needed protection for infants and small children for whom normal restraints do not work adequately by themselves because of the children's rapidly changing anatomical dimensions. The seat faces rearward for infants and very small children, then should be turned to face forward as the child grows. This positioning permits the seat belt to provide restraint, similar to that provided for the adult. Child safety seats should not be positioned in front of airbag restraint systems because inflation of those devices may push the rear-facing child forcibly into the seat.

Motorcycle helmet use can significantly reduce the incidence and severity of head injury, the greatest cause of motorcycle crash death. Helmets do not, however, reduce the incidence of spinal injury.

5. Describe the mechanisms of injury associated with falls, crush injuries, and sports injuries.   pp. 49–52

Falls are a release of stored gravitational energy resulting in an impact between the body and the ground or other surface. Injuries occur at the point of impact and along the pathway of transmitted energy, resulting in soft tissue, skeletal, and internal trauma.

Crush injuries are injuries caused by heavy objects or machinery entrapping and damaging an extremity. The resulting wound restricts blood flow and allows the accumulation of toxins. When the pressure is removed, blood flow may move the toxins into the central circulation and hemorrhage from many disrupted blood vessels at the wound site may be hard to control.

Sports injuries are commonly the result of direct trauma, fatigue, or exertion. They often result in injury to muscles, ligaments, and tendons and to the long bones. Special consideration must be given to protecting such an injury from further aggravation until it can be seen by a physician.

6. Identify the common blast injuries and any special considerations regarding their assessment and proper care.   pp. 42–49

The blast injury process results in five distinct mechanisms of injury—pressure injury, penetrating objects, personnel displacement, structural collapse, and burns.

Pressure injury occurs as the pressure wave moves outward, rapidly compressing, then decompressing anything in its path. A victim is impacted by the wave and air-filled body spaces such as the lungs, auditory canals, and bowels may be damaged. Hearing loss is the most frequent result of pressure injury, though lung injury is most serious and life threatening. The pressure change may damage or rupture alveoli resulting in dyspnea, pulmonary edema, pneumothorax, or air embolism. Care includes provision of high-flow oxygen, gentle positive-pressure ventilation, and rapid transport. The hearing loss patient needs careful reassurance and simple instruction.

Penetrating objects may be the bomb casing or debris put in motion by the pressure of the explosion. They may impale or enter the body, resulting in hemorrhage and internal injury. Care specific to the resulting injury should be provided, and any hemorrhage controlled by direct pressure. Any impaled object should be immobilized and the patient given rapid transport to the trauma center.

Personnel displacement occurs as the pressure wave and blast wind propel the victim through the air and he or she then impacts the ground or other surface. Blunt and penetrating trauma may result, and such injuries are cared for following standard procedures.

Collapse of a structure after a blast may entrap victims under debris and result in crush and pressure injuries. The collapse may make victims hard to locate and then extricate. Further, the nature of the crush-type wounds may make control of hemorrhage difficult, while the release of a long-entrapped extremity may be dangerous as the toxins that accumulated when circulation is disrupted are distributed to the central circulation.

Burns may result directly from the explosion or as a result of secondary combustion of debris or clothing. Generally the initial explosion will cause only superficial damage because of the short duration of the heat release and the fluid nature of the body. However, incendiary agents and burning debris or clothing may result in severe full-thickness burns.

7. Identify and explain any special assessment and care considerations for patients with blunt trauma. pp. 28–52

Blunt injury patients must be carefully assessed because the signs of serious internal injury may be hidden or absent. Careful analysis of the mechanism of injury and the development of an index of suspicion for serious injury may be the only way to anticipate the true seriousness of the injuries.

8. Given several scenarios involving simulated blunt trauma patients, provide the appropriate scene size-up, initial assessment, focused assessment, detailed assessment, and then provide appropriate patient care and transportation. pp. 28–52

During your training as an EMT-Paramedic, you will participate in many classroom practice sessions involving simulated patients. You will also spend some time in the emergency departments of local hospitals as well as in advanced-level ambulances gaining clinical experience. During these times, use your knowledge of the mechanisms of blunt trauma to help you assess and care for the simulated or real patients you attend.

CASE STUDY REVIEW

Reread the case study on pages 17, 18, and 19 in Paramedic Care: Trauma Emergencies *before reading the discussion below.*

This scenario represents a typical serious auto collision in which knowledge of the kinetics of trauma assists in analyzing the mechanism of injury and helps guide assessment and care. Using this approach results in a better understanding of the potential injuries. It also provides for an orderly scene approach in which the patients are quickly assessed, prioritized, immediately stabilized, and then quickly transported. The incident is evaluated carefully, using an analysis of the mechanism of injury to anticipate both the nature and severity of patient injuries. This information is then used in combination with the data gathered through the patient assessments to develop a clear picture of what happened to the auto passengers and to determine what resources will be distributed to each patient.

The information given by the dispatcher allows Kris and Bob to begin planning for arrival at the scene. The dispatch information describes a severe accident with the potential for several seriously injured patients. While still en route, Kris and Bob locate equipment in the ambulance and set it out on the stretcher for quick transport to their patients' side. Lactated Ringer's solution in 1,000 mL bags might be readied in the ambulance with trauma tubing, pressure infusers, and large-bore catheters readied, just in case the decision is made to rapidly transport the patient. Kris and Bob may also use this time to review their responsibilities, which begin with arrival at the scene.

Given the police update, the team begins thinking about the kinetic energy associated with the collision and the injuries that it is likely to cause. One auto was stopped and was hit from behind by a vehicle at "highway speed." In the auto hit, the suspected injuries should include cervical spine injury, with the rest of the body well protected except for secondary impacts. Kris and Bob should anticipate the need for spinal precautions and ready a collar, vest-type immobilization device, and long spine board.

The auto traveling at highway speed most likely impacted the other frontally. If the occupants were unrestrained, they may have traveled either through the down-and-under or up-and-over pathway. If they were restrained, the lap, lap and shoulder, or airbag restraint systems may have protected them. (Remember that the airbag restraint system is beneficial only for the initial frontal impact.) Internal head injuries, chest trauma, and shock are the leading trauma killers. The team will anticipate these types of injuries and treat their patients accordingly.

Kris and Bob gain a great deal of information quickly during the scene size-up. Potential hazards, the number of patients, the resources needed, and the mechanism of injury all are identified. From analysis of the mechanism of injury, they anticipate the nature and extent of injuries for each of the three expected patients. By examining what happened, how badly the autos are damaged, and from what direction the impacts came, the team can garner enough information to anticipate which patient is likely to be the most seriously injured.

In this collision, the green car struck the red one from behind. The red car sustained severe rear-end damage, reflecting a strong impact. The passenger would have been pushed forward with great acceleration by the auto seat, while the unsupported head rotated backward, extending the cervical spine. An important observation was that the headrest was in the "up" position. This positioning probably limited the forceful hyperextension of the head and neck and reduced the potential for injury. The seatbelt also limited the danger of secondary impact, assuring the driver came to rest with the vehicle, not afterward.

The second car (the green one) sustained front-end damage and two spider-web cracks in the windshield. This suggests an unrestrained driver and passenger, the up-and-over pathway, and a potential for severe head, neck, thoracic, and abdominal injuries. The deformed steering wheel also provides evidence that the driver may have sustained a chest injury. Using the analysis of the mechanism of injury, Kris and Bob have a good preliminary picture of the collision process and the likely injuries it produced. As they leave their vehicle and approach the scene, they don gloves and assure the scene is safe for them, their patients, fellow rescuers, and bystanders. They also request anticipated resources (another ambulance) to handle the multiple patients they expect. Because the mechanism of injury analysis suggests the most serious patients will be found in the green car, Kris and Bob head there first.

Assessment confirms the injuries anticipated by review of the impact and the degree of auto damage. As reported by the police officer, the driver of the red car appears only shaken up with a possible spine injury. His vitals are within normal limits, given the circumstances. The choice is made to leave him with a First Responder while Kris and Bob remain with the patients in the green car. While it would be more preferable to have a paramedic by the side of each patient, this decision is justified based upon the findings at the scene. Bob and Kris will have another First Responder hold spinal immobilization for the driver of the green car as they attend to the unconscious passenger.

The initial assessment reveals that the occupants of the green auto are in serious condition. The driver has sustained chest trauma and is experiencing dyspnea, though her breath sounds are clear at this time. She is stable for now. However, she has the potential to deteriorate rapidly at any time. Her passenger is moving rapidly into hypovolemic shock, presumably due to pelvic and femur fractures and internal hemorrhage. She is also unconscious either due to the hypovolemia or the head impact. The passenger is critical and a candidate for immediate transport. The driver, though more stable, is a candidate for immediate transport also.

This case study demonstrates the value a good scene analysis can have in triaging, in anticipating the findings of assessment, and in determining the care needed by the patient or patients. While the mechanism of injury analysis does not give definitive information regarding the nature and extent of patient injuries, it can complement the overall assessment of both the scene and each individual patient.

CONTENT SELF-EVALUATION

MULTIPLE CHOICE

_____ 1. The study of trauma is related to a branch of physics called:
A. kinetics.
B. velocity.
C. ballistics.
D. inertia.
E. heuristics.

_____ 2. The anticipation of injuries based upon the analysis of the collision mechanism is referred to as the:
A. mechanism of injury.
B. index of suspicion.
C. trauma triage criteria.
D. mortality potential.
E. RTS.

_____ 3. Penetrating trauma is the most common type of trauma associated with patient mortality.
A. True
B. False

_____ 4. The tendency of an object to remain at rest or remain in motion unless acted upon by an external force is:
A. kinetics.
B. velocity.
C. ballistics.
D. inertia.
E. deceleration.

_____ 5. Two autos accelerate from a stop sign to a speed of 30 mph, the first one by normal acceleration and the second when it was struck from behind by another vehicle. Assuming that both vehicles have the same weight, which vehicle gained the most kinetic energy?
A. the vehicle in normal acceleration
B. the vehicle struck from behind
C. both vehicles gained the same kinetic energy
D. cannot be determined since the kinetic energy is not known
E. cannot be determined since the force is not known

_____ 6. Which of the following is an example of energy dissipation from an auto accident?
A. sound of the impact
B. bending of the structural steel
C. heating of the compressed steel
D. internal injury to the occupant
E. all of the above

_____ 7. Which of the following increases the kinetic energy of a collision most quickly?
A. the temperature of the object
B. increasing object speed
C. decreasing object speed
D. increasing object mass
E. decreasing object mass

_____ 8. Blunt trauma may cause:
A. rupture of the bowel.
B. bursting of the alveoli.
C. crushing of blood vessels.
D. contusion of the liver or kidneys.
E. all of the above.

_____ 9. Which of the following is a common cause of blunt trauma?
A. auto collisions
B. falls
C. sports injuries
D. pedestrian impacts
E. all of the above

_____ 10. In which order do the events of an auto collision usually occur?
A. body collision, vehicle collision, organ collision, secondary collisions
B. organ collision, vehicle collision, body collision, secondary collisions
C. vehicle collision, secondary collisions, body collision, organ collision
D. vehicle collision, body collision, organ collision, secondary collisions
E. body collision, vehicle collision, secondary collisions, organ collision

_____ 11. The major effect of the seat belt during the auto collision is to slow the passenger with the auto.
   A. True
   B. False

_____ 12. A supplemental restraint system (SRS) refers to which of the following?
   A. shoulder belts   D. child seats
   B. airbags   E. all of the above
   C. lap belts

_____ 13. Which of the following restraint systems is likely to induce hand fractures?
   A. shoulder belts   D. child seats
   B. passenger airbags   E. lap belts
   C. driver-side airbags

_____ 14. While less convenient than a child carrier, holding a child in the arms is relatively safe except in the most severe of crashes.
   A. True
   B. False

_____ 15. The type of auto impact that occurs most frequently in rural areas is:
   A. lateral.   D. rear-end.
   B. rotational.   E. rollover.
   C. frontal.

_____ 16. Which type of auto impact occurs most frequently in the urban setting?
   A. lateral   D. rear-end
   B. rotational   E. rollover
   C. frontal

_____ 17. The down-and-under pathway is most commonly associated with which type of auto collision?
   A. lateral   D. rear-end
   B. rotational   E. rollover
   C. frontal

_____ 18. When analyzing the lateral impact injury mechanism, you must assign a higher index of suspicion for serious life-threatening injury than with other types of impact.
   A. True
   B. False

_____ 19. Which of the following injuries are associated with significant lateral impact?
   A. aortic aneurysms   D. vertebral fractures
   B. clavicular fractures E. all of the above
   C. pelvic fractures

_____ 20. With rotational impacts, the seriousness of injury is often less than vehicle damage would suggest.
   A. True
   B. False

_____ 21. The most common injury associated with the rear-end impact is to the:
   A. abdomen.   D. femur.
   B. pelvis.   E. head and neck.
   C. aorta.

_____ 22. Which of the following is a hazard commonly associated with auto collisions?
   A. hot liquids   D. sharp glass or metal edges
   B. caustic substances   E. all of the above
   C. downed power lines

_____ 23. With modern vehicle construction that incorporates crumple zones, you can dependably use the amount of vehicular damage to approximate the patient injuries inside.
   A. True
   B. False

_____ 24. In fatal collisions, about what percentage of the drivers are legally intoxicated?
   A. 10 percent   D. 50 percent
   B. 20 percent   E. 83 percent
   C. 35 percent

_____ 25. The most common body area associated with vehicular mortality is the:
   A. head.   D. extremities.
   B. chest.   E. spine.
   C. abdomen.

_____ 26. In motorcycle accidents, the highest index of suspicion for injury should be directed at the:
   A. neck.   D. pelvis.
   B. head.   E. femurs.
   C. extremities.

_____ 27. Use of a helmet in a motorcycle crash reduces the incidence of neck injury by about:
   A. 25 percent.   D. 75 percent.
   B. 35 percent.   E. 85 percent.
   C. 58 percent.

_____ 28. In an auto vs. child pedestrian accident, you would expect the victim to turn toward the impact.
   A. True
   B. False

_____ 29. In addition to the danger of trauma, the boating collision patient is also likely to suffer possible hypothermia and near-drowning.
   A. True
   B. False

_____ 30. Which of the mechanisms below can cause patient injury in a blast?
   A. the pressure wave
   B. flying debris
   C. the patient being thrown into objects
   D. heat
   E. all of the above

_____ 31. Underwater detonation of an explosive generally increases its lethal range by:
   A. 10 percent.   D. 300 percent.
   B. 25 percent.   E. 500 percent.
   C. 100 percent.

_____ 32. A victim's orientation to the blast does not effect the nature and severity of the injuries he or she sustains from an explosion.
   A. True
   B. False

_____ 33. The arrow-shaped projectiles in military-type explosives that are designed to extend the injury power of a bomb are called:
   A. ordinance.   D. oatmeal.
   B. casing material.   E. granulation.
   C. flechettes.

_____ 34. When victims are within a structure that contains an explosion, like a building, the effects of the blast are concentrated and the severity of the expected injuries increases.
   A. True
   B. False

_____ 35. Which of the following are secondary blast injuries?
A. heat injuries
B. pressure injuries
C. projectile injuries
D. injuries caused by structural collapse
E. both A and B

_____ 36. If you suspect that a blast was a terrorist act, you should be cautious of secondary explosive devices intended to injure rescue personnel.
A. True
B. False

_____ 37. The most serious and common traumas associated with explosions affect the:
A. heart.
B. bowel.
C. auditory canal.
D. lungs.
E. brain.

_____ 38. When ventilating the victim of a severe blast, you should use forceful deep ventilations with the bag-valve mask as doing this will assure good chest expansion.
A. True
B. False

_____ 39. Severe injury is generally associated with a fall from:
A. three times the patient's own height.
B. twice the patient's own height.
C. greater than 12 feet.
D. more than 6 feet.
E. none of the above

_____ 40. Sports injuries are frequently associated with:
A. fatigue.
B. extreme exertion.
C. compression.
D. rotation.
E. all of the above

SPECIAL PROJECT

Mechanism of Injury Analysis

Study the photographs of each accident scene below. For each photo, identify the type of impact that has occurred and list at least three injuries that you would expect to have occurred.

A. Mechanism of injury _____

Anticipated injuries

_____

_____

_____

_____

_____

_____

_____

_____

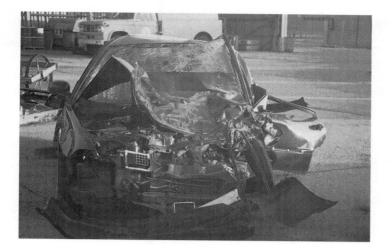

B. Mechanism of injury _____

Anticipated injuries

_____

_____

_____

_____

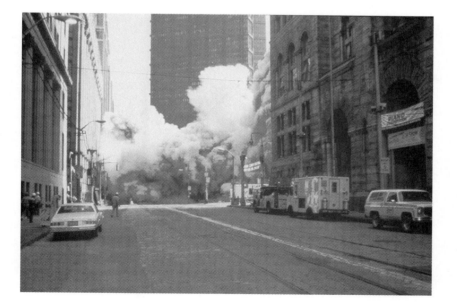

C. Mechanism of injury _____

Anticipated injuries

_____

_____

_____

_____

Personal Benchmarking—Analyzing Mechanisms of Injury

Next time you are in a vehicle for some time, take a look at your position with regard to the interior of the auto in relation to your anatomy. Visualize the forces of impact and what your body will strike during that impact. Identify protections offered by crumple zones and the likely injuries resulting from serious impact, and then determine what effect restraints will have on injury patterns (nature and seriousness).

Frontal Impact

Lateral Impact

Rear-end Impact

Rotational Impact

Rollover Impact

The next time you go to an auto collision, use this information to help you "relive" the auto impact and anticipate patient injuries.

CHAPTER 3
*

Penetrating Trauma

Review of Chapter Objectives

After reading this chapter, you should be able to:

1. **Explain the energy exchange process between a penetrating object or projectile and the object it strikes.**   pp. 57–61

The kinetic energy of a bullet is dependent upon its mass and even more so on its velocity according to the kinetic energy formula (KE = $\frac{M \times V^2}{2}$). This energy is distributed to the body tissues in the form of damage as the bullet slows. Due to the semifluid nature of body tissue, the passage of a bullet causes injury as the bullet directly strikes tissue and contuses and tears it and as it sets the tissue in motion outward and away from the bullet's path (cavitation). The faster the bullet and the larger its presenting surface (profile), the more rapid the exchange of energy and the resulting injury.

2. **Determine the effects profile, yaw, tumble, expansion, and fragmentation have on projectile energy transfer.**   pp. 58–61

The rate of projectile energy exchange and the seriousness of resulting injury are dependent upon the rate of energy exchange. That rate is directly related to the bullet's presenting surface or profile. The larger the bullet's caliber (diameter), the greater its profile, the more rapid its exchange of energy with body tissue, and the greater the damage it causes. Yaw (swinging around the axis of the projectile's travel), tumble, expansion, and fragmentation all lead to a greater area of the bullet striking tissue than simply its profile, and hence these factors increase the damaging power of a bullet.

3. **Describe elements of the ballistic injury process including direct injury, cavitation, temporary cavity, permanent cavity, and zone of injury.**   pp. 58–61, 64–67

As a penetrating object enters the body it disrupts the tissue it contacts by tearing it, displacing it from its path, and causing *direct injury*. As the object's velocity increases, the rate of energy exchange increases and the rate of displacement increases. A bullet's speed is so great that the bullet's passage sets the semifluid body tissue in motion away from the bullet's path. This creates a cavity behind and to the side of the projectile pathway. This *cavitation* further stretches and tears tissue as it creates a *temporary cavity*. The natural elasticity of injured tissue and the adjoining tissue closes the cavity, but an area of disrupted tissue remains (the *permanent cavity*). The *zone of injury* is the region along and surrounding the bullet track where tissue has been disrupted due to direct injury or to the stretching and tearing of cavitation.

4. **Identify the relative effects a penetrating object or projectile has when striking various body regions and tissues.**   pp. 67–71

The passage of a bullet (and its cavitational wave) has varying effects depending on the elasticity (resiliency) and density of the tissue the bullet strikes. Connective tissue is very resilient, stretches easily, and will somewhat resist cavitational injury. Solid organs are generally very dense and much less resilient than connective tissue. They do not withstand the force generated by the cavitational wave as well as connective tissue, and the resulting injury can be expected to be much greater. Hollow organs are resilient when not distended with fluid; if an organ is full, however, the cavitational wave may cause the organ to rupture. Direct injury can also perforate an organ and permit spillage of its contents into surrounding tissue. Lung tissue is both very resilient and air filled. The tiny air pockets (the alveoli) absorb the energy of the bullet's passage and limit lung injury. On the other hand, bone is extremely dense and inelastic. Direct contact with a bullet or, in some cases, just the cavitational wave may shatter the bone and drive fragments into surrounding tissue. Slow-moving penetrating objects do not produce a cavitational wave, and injury from them is limited to the pathway of the object.

The passage of a bullet and its associated injury are related to the bullet's path of travel and, specifically, to the body region it passes through. Extremity wounds are by far the most common, yet due to the limited major body structures in the extremities, they rarely result in life-threatening injury. If the projectile strikes the bone, however, the dramatic exchange of energy may cause great tissue disruption and vascular injury, which can result in severe hemorrhage. Abdominal penetration most commonly affects the bowel, which is reasonably tolerant of the cavitational wave. However, the upper abdomen contains the liver, pancreas, and spleen, solid organs that are subject to severe injury from direct injury and cavitation. Penetrating chest trauma may affect the lungs, heart and great vessels, esophagus, trachea, and diaphragm. The lung is rather resilient to penetrating injury, while the heart and great vessels may perforate or rupture with rapid exsanguination ensuing. Tracheal tears may result in airway compromise, while esophageal tears may release gastric contents into the mediastinum with potentially deadly results. Large penetrations of the thoracic wall may permit air to move in and out (sucking or open pneumothorax) or may open the airway internally to permit air to enter the pleural space (closed pneumothorax). Neck injuries may permit severe hemorrhage, disrupt the trachea, or allow air to enter the jugular veins and embolize the lungs. Head injuries may disrupt the airway or may penetrate the cranium and cause extensive, rarely survivable, injury to the brain.

5. **Anticipate the injury types and extent of damage associated with high-velocity/high-energy projectiles, such as rifle bullets; with medium velocity/medium-energy projectiles, such as handgun and shotgun bullets, slugs, or pellets; and with low-energy/low-velocity penetrating objects, such as knives and arrows.** pp. 61–64

High-velocity/high-energy projectiles (rifle bullets) are likely to cause the most extensive injury because they have the potential to impart the most kinetic energy to the patient. Their rapid energy exchange causes the greatest cavitational wave and is most likely to produce bullet deformity and fragmentation. These characteristics cause more severe tissue damage to a greater area. The effects of these projectiles can be further enhanced if the bullet hits bone and causes it to shatter, creating additional projectiles that are driven into adjoining tissue.

Medium-velocity/medium-energy projectiles (from handguns) are likely to cause only moderate injury beyond the direct pathway of the bullet as their reduced energy does not usually cause the bullet deformity, fragmentation, and extensive cavitation waves seen with rifle projectiles. The shotgun is a particularly lethal weapon at close range because its medium-energy projectiles are numerous and their numbers cause many direct injury pathways.

Low-velocity/low-energy penetrating objects are commonly knives, arrows, ice picks, and other objects traveling at low speeds. They generally cause only direct injury along the path of their travel. They may, however, be moved about, once inserted and either left in place or withdrawn.

6. **Identify important elements of the scene size-up associated with shootings or stabbings.** pp. 72–73

Penetrating trauma, especially when associated with shootings or stabbings, presents the danger of violence directed toward others (other rescuers, bystanders, your patient, and you). It is essential that you approach the scene with great caution and ensure that the police have secured it before you approach or enter. Penetrating trauma also calls for gloves as minimum BSI precaution, with goggles and gown required for spurting hemorrhage, airway management, or massive blood contamination. During the scene size-up, you should evaluate the mechanism of injury including the type of weapon, caliber, distance, and angle between the shooter and the victim, and the number of shots fired and patient impacts.

7. Identify and explain any special assessment and care considerations for patients with penetrating trauma. pp. 73–74

In assessing the patient with penetrating trauma you must anticipate the projectile or penetrating object's pathway and the structures it is likely to have injured. The exit wound from a projectile may help you better approximate the wounding potential, and remember that the bullet may have been deflected along its course and damaged or completely missed critical structures. Always suspect and treat for the worst-case scenario. Be especially wary of injuries to the head, chest, and abdomen as wounds to these regions often have lethal outcomes. Cover all open wounds that enter the thorax or neck with occlusive dressings and be watchful for the development of dyspnea due to pneumothorax, tension pneumothorax, or pulmonary emboli. Be prepared to provide aggressive fluid resuscitation, but understand that doing so may dislodge forming clots and increase the rate of internal hemorrhage. Stabilize any impaled objects and only remove them when it is required to assure a patent airway, to perform CPR, or to transport the patient.

8. Presented with several preprogrammed situations involving simulated penetrating trauma patients, provide the appropriate scene size-up, initial assessment, focused history and detailed physical exam, and ongoing assessment, and then provide appropriate patient care and transportation. pp. 57–74

During your training as an EMT-Paramedic you will participate in many classroom practice sessions involving simulated patients. You will also spend some time in the emergency departments of local hospitals as well as in advanced-level ambulances gaining clinical experience. During these times, use your knowledge of the mechanisms of penetrating trauma to help you assess and care for the simulated or real patients you attend.

CASE STUDY REVIEW

Reread the case study on pages 55 and 56 in Paramedic Care: Trauma Emergencies *before reading the discussion below.*

This scenario involves a patient who has sustained a serious penetrating injury to the chest and provides the opportunity to apply an understanding of the kinetics of trauma to the wounding process. The case also allows us to review scene considerations that should be followed when violence is involved.

Weapon use in modern society represents violence and a danger to rescuers, bystanders, the patient, and the responding EMS team. Sandy is somewhat reassured by the dispatch information, which states that the victim is in custody, and more so as she arrives at the scene and notes the police officers surrounding the patient. However, she remains cautious and ensures that the victim is free of weapons before she begins her care.

In assessing the patient, Sandy anticipates a serious injury, as police are generally equipped with relatively powerful handguns. She recognizes that the bullet delivered significant wounding energy to the thorax and may have fragmented as it hit the ribs and drove rib fragments into tissue as it passed. She anticipates lung damage along the bullet's path, probably more related to the damage seen at the exit, rather than at the entrance, wound. Sandy is also concerned about the penetration of the chest wall and the pleura caused by the bullet's passage. Such a wound may permit air to enter the pleural space and cause the lung to collapse (an open pneumothorax). She seals both the entrance and exit wounds on three sides to allow any building air pressure (tension pneumothorax) to escape. She also carefully monitors breath sounds and respiratory effort to assure an unrecognized close tension pneumothorax does not develop. Sandy anticipates that this patient's respirations will worsen as the edema associated with the injured lung tissue gets worse and with the continued loss of blood from the internal wound.

Due to the proximity of the wound to the heart, Sandy applies the ECG electrodes and constantly monitors the patient's heart rate and rhythm. She also trends both the patient's level of consciousness and vital signs to assure that the earliest signs of hypovolemia, shock, and decreased tissue perfusion are noted. This patient is clearly a candidate for rapid transport to the closest trauma center.

CONTENT SELF-EVALUATION

MULTIPLE CHOICE

_____ 1. Approximately what number of deaths are attributable to shootings each year?
A. 25,000
B. 38,000
C. 44,000
D. 50,000
E. 100,000

_____ 2. An object traveling at twice the speed of another object of the same weight has:
A. twice the kinetic energy.
B. three times the kinetic energy.
C. four times the kinetic energy.
D. eight times the kinetic energy.
E. ten times the kinetic energy.

_____ 3. Wounds from rifle bullets are considered two to four times more lethal handgun bullets.
A. True
B. False

_____ 4. The curved tract a bullet follows during flight is called its:
A. ballistics.
B. cavitation.
C. trajectory.
D. yaw.
E. parabola.

_____ 5. The surface of a projectile that exchanges energy with the object struck is its:
A. caliber.
B. profile.
C. drag.
D. yaw.
E. expansion factor.

_____ 6. When a rifle bullet hits tissue, normally it will:
A. continue without tumbling.
B. tumble once then travel nose first.
C. tumble quickly, the slowly rotate.
D. wobble but not tumble.
E. tumble 180 degrees then continue.

_____ 7. Because handgun bullets are made of relatively soft lead, their kinetic energy is generally not sufficient to cause significant deformity.
A. True
B. False

_____ 8. Civilian hunting ammunition is designed to deform and will frequently fragment when striking soft tissue.
A. True
B. False

_____ 9. Which of the following statements accurately describes a rifle bullet in contrast to a handgun bullet?
A. It is a heavier projectile.
B. It travels at a greater velocity.
C. It is more likely to deform.
D. It is more likely to fragment.
E. all of the above

_____ 10. The shotgun is limited in range and accuracy; however, injuries it inflicts at close range can be very severe or lethal.
A. True
B. False

_____ 11. Which element of the projectile injury process is related to the actual damage caused as the bullet contacts tissue?
   A. direct injury
   B. pressure wave
   C. temporary cavity
   D. permanent cavity
   E. zone of injury

_____ 12. The formation of sub-atmospheric pressure behind the bullet as it passes through the body results in:
   A. direct injury.
   B. the pressure wave.
   C. a temporary cavity.
   D. fragmentation.
   E. referred injury.

_____ 13. The passage of a projectile through the body results in a region where tissues are disrupted and not functioning normally that is known as the:
   A. direct injury.
   B. pressure wave.
   C. temporary cavity.
   D. permanent cavity.
   E. zone of injury.

_____ 14. The temporary cavity formed as a high-velocity/high-energy bullet passes may be how large?
   A. 2 times the bullet caliber
   B. 4 times the bullet caliber
   C. 6 times the bullet caliber
   D. 10 times the bullet caliber
   E. rarely more than the bullet caliber

_____ 15. The tissue structure that is very resilient, yet dense, and usually sustains limited damage with the passage of a projectile is:
   A. a solid organ.
   B. a hollow organ.
   C. connective tissue.
   D. bone.
   E. a lung.

_____ 16. The tissue structure that is likely to rupture and spill its contents when struck by a projectile is:
   A. a solid organ.
   B. a hollow organ.
   C. connective tissue.
   D. bone.
   E. a lung.

_____ 17. Penetrating wounds to the extremities account for about 70 percent of all penetrating wounds yet account for less than 10 percent of fatalities related to this injury mechanism.
   A. True
   B. False

_____ 18. The abdominal organ most tolerant to the passage of a projectile is the:
   A. bowel.
   B. liver.
   C. spleen.
   D. kidney.
   E. pancreas.

_____ 19. Because of the pressure-driven dynamics of respiration, any large wound to the chest may compromise breathing.
   A. True
   B. False

_____ 20. The body region in which a penetrating wound has the greatest likelihood of drawing air into the venous system is the:
   A. abdomen.
   B. thorax.
   C. head.
   D. neck.
   E. none of the above

_____ 21. Which of the following is NOT associated with an entrance wound?
   A. tattooing
   B. a small ridge of discoloration around the wound
   C. a blown outward appearance
   D. subcutaneous emphysema
   E. propellant residue on the surrounding tissue

_____ 22. The entrance wound is more likely to reflect the actual damaging potential of the projectile than the exit wound.
   A. True
   B. False

_____ 23. Which of the following information should you gain through the scene size-up, if possible?
   A. the gun caliber
   B. the angle of the gun to the victim
   C. the type of gun used
   D. assurance that no other weapons are involved
   E. all of the above

_____ 24. As you care for a patient at a potential crime scene, actions you take to help preserve evidence should include:
   A. cutting through, not around bullet or knife holes in clothing.
   B. moving what you can away from the patient.
   C. removing obviously dead patients from the scene as quickly as possible.
   D. disturbing only the items necessary to provide patient care.
   E. all of the above

_____ 25. Frothy blood at a bullet exit or entrance wound suggests a(n):
   A. simple pneumothorax.   D. pericardial tamponade.
   B. open pneumothorax.   E. mediastinum injury.
   C. tension pneumothorax.

SPECIAL PROJECT

Label the Diagram

Demonstrate your knowledge of the process by which projectiles injure body tissue by identifying the labels A through E on the diagram below showing a bullet's penetration of the body.

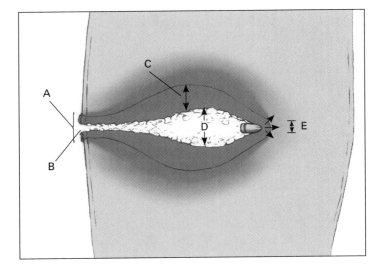

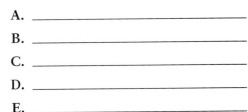

A. _____

B. _____

C. _____

D. _____

E. _____

CHAPTER 4
*
Hemorrhage and Shock

Review of Chapter Objectives

After reading this chapter, you should be able to:

1. **Describe the epidemiology, including the morbidity/mortality and prevention strategies, for shock and hemorrhage.**   pp. 89–91, 99–108

   Shock is the transitional stage between normal physiologic function of the body and death. It is the underlying killer of all trauma patients and is prevented using the strategies described for each of the types of trauma addressed by the following seven chapters. Hemorrhage is loss of the body's precious medium, blood, and is a common cause of shock and death in the trauma patient. Strategies to prevent hemorrhage are those designed to prevent trauma as discussed in the next seven chapters.

2. **Discuss the anatomy, physiology, and pathophysiology of the cardiovascular system as they apply to hemorrhage and shock.**   pp. 79–82, 99–108

   The cardiovascular system is a closed system of interconnected tubes (blood vessels) that direct blood to the essential organs and tissues of the body. Arteries distribute blood to the various organs and tissues of the body. Arterioles determine the amount of blood perfusing the tissue of an organ and together constrict and increase peripheral vascular resistance or dilate and reduce peripheral vascular resistance. Progressive vasoconstriction can help maintain blood pressure and circulation to the most critical organs as the body loses blood during hemorrhage or fluid during other forms of shock. The venous system collects blood and returns it to the heart. It contains about 60 percent of the total blood volume and, when constricted, can return a relatively great volume (up to 1 liter) to the active circulation.

   The cardiovascular system is powered by the central pump, the heart. It circulates the blood and, against the peripheral vascular resistance, drives the blood pressure. Its output is a factor of preload (the blood delivered to it by the venous system), stroke volume (the amount of blood ejected into the aorta with each contraction), rate, and afterload (the peripheral vascular resistance). The heart can help compensate for blood loss by attempting to maintain cardiac output by increasing its stroke volume (which is hard to do in hypovolemic states) or by increasing its rate.

   Finally, the cardiovascular system contains the precious fluid, blood. Blood provides oxygen and nutrients to the body cells and removes carbon dioxide and waste products of metabolism. Blood also contains clotting factors that will occlude blood vessels if they are torn or disrupted.

   The central nervous system provides control of the cardiovascular system using baroreceptors in the carotid arteries and aortic arch to sense fluctuations in blood pressure. It will maintain blood pressure by increasing heart rate, cardiac preload, and peripheral vascular resistance. Hormones from the kidneys and elsewhere help control blood volume and electrolytes as well as the production of erythrocytes.

3. **Define shock based on aerobic and anaerobic metabolism.** pp. 99–101

Cells are the elemental building blocks of the body and ultimately carry out all body functions. They derive their energy from a two-step process. The first step, called glycolysis, requires no oxygen (anaerobic) and generates a small amount of energy. The second step, called the citric acid or Krebs cycle, requires oxygen (aerobic) and generates about 95 percent of the cell's energy. In shock, which is inadequate tissue perfusion that does not adequately supply the cells with oxygen, the cells produce energy in an inefficient way and toxins accumulate.

4. **Describe the body's physiologic response to changes in blood volume, blood pressure, and perfusion.** pp. 99–112

Increased peripheral resistance is caused by the constriction of the arterioles and provides two mechanisms that combat shock. The arterioles constrict and maintain the blood pressure, and they divert blood to only the critical organs. This reduction in perfusion to the less critical organs results in the increased capillary refill time and the cool, clammy, and ashen skin often associated with shock states. It also results in reduced pulse pressure and weak pulses.

Venous constriction compensates for some blood loss and helps maintain cardiac preload. Since the veins account for about 60 percent of the blood volume, this is reasonably effective in minor to moderate blood loss.

As the cardiac preload drops, the heart rate increases in an attempt to maintain cardiac output and blood pressure. In the presence of significantly reduced preload, this may not be effective.

Peripheral vascular shunting directs the blood away from the skin, conserves body heat, and reduces fluid loss through evaporation. It also redirects blood to more critical areas.

Fluid shifts are the result of drawing fluid from the interstitial and cellular spaces. Fluid moves into the vascular space. While this is a slow mechanism, it can provide the vascular system with several liters of fluid.

5. **Describe the effects of decreased perfusion at the capillary level.** pp. 101–104, 107–108

Decreased capillary perfusion limits the amount of oxygen and nutrients delivered to the body cells. It usually causes the release of histamine that, in turn, causes precapillary sphincter dilation and an increase in perfusion. However, in shock states this is not effective, and the cells must revert to anaerobic metabolism while the byproducts of metabolism accumulate and the available oxygen is exhausted. Carbon dioxide, metabolic acids, and other waste products accumulate while body cells begin to die.

6. **Discuss the cellular ischemic, capillary stagnation, and capillary washout phases related to hemorrhagic shock.** pp. 107–108

Ischemia. As shock ensues, decreased perfusion, first to the non-critical organs, then to all organs, diminishes blood flow through the microcirculation. At the cellular level this diminishes the supply of oxygen and nutrients to the cells and restricts the removal of carbon dioxide and the waste products of metabolism. The cells quickly exhaust their supply of oxygen and begin to use anaerobic metabolism as their sole source of energy to remain alive. This produces an accumulation of pyruvic acid, which in turn, converts to lactic acid and the cells become more acidotic. As cells begin to die, their decomposition releases even more toxins that then begin to affect other cells.

Capillary stagnation. With diminished capillary flow, coupled with the increasingly hypoxic and acidic environment caused by the ischemic cells, the red blood cells become sticky and clump together. They form columns of coagulated erythrocytes called rouleaux that either block the capillary to further flow of blood or will wash out and cause microemboli.

Capillary washout. The toxic environment of the ischemic tissue associated with severe shock finally causes the post-capillary sphincters to dilate and release the hypoxic and acidotic blood as well as the rouleaux into the venous circulation. As this washout becomes extensive, it further reduces the effectiveness of the cardiovascular system and the body moves quickly toward irreversible shock.

7. **Discuss the various types and degrees of shock and hemorrhage.** **pp. 89–93, 108–110**

Hemorrhage can be divided into four stages as a patient moves through compensated, decompensated, and irreversible shock.

Stage 1 blood loss is a loss of up to 15 percent of the patient's blood volume. It generally presents with some nervousness, cool skin, and slight pallor. It is difficult to detect as the body compensates well for blood loss in this range.

Stage 2 blood loss is a loss of up to 25 percent of the patient's blood volume. Signs and symptoms become more apparent as the body finds it more difficult to compensate for the loss. The patient may display thirst, anxiety, restlessness, and cool and clammy skin.

Stage 3 blood loss is a loss of up to 35 percent of the patient's blood volume. It presents with the signs of stage 2 blood loss and air hunger, dyspnea, and severe thirst. Survival is unlikely without immediate intervention.

Stage 4 blood loss is a blood loss in excess of 35 percent of the patient's blood volume. The patient begins to display a deathlike appearance with pulses disappearing and respirations becoming very shallow and ineffective. The patient becomes very lethargic and then unconscious and survival becomes unlikely.

8. **Predict shock and hemorrhage based on mechanism of injury.** **pp. 92–93, 112**

Shock due to internal blood loss can be a very silent killer if not recognized and the patient brought to definitive care (surgery) quickly. Severe blunt and deep penetrating trauma can induce internal hemorrhage that is both difficult to identify and treat. If you wait until the frank signs of shock appear, too much time may have passed for care to be effective. Hence it is very important to both analyze the mechanism of injury to anticipate shock and to recognize the very early signs of shock.

A large hematoma may account for up to 500 mL of blood loss, while fractures of the humerus or tibia/fibula may account for 500 to 750 mL. Femoral fractures may account for up to 1,500 mL of blood, while pelvic fractures often involve hemorrhage of up to 2,000 mL. Internal hemorrhage into the chest or abdomen may contribute even greater losses. In penetrating or severe blunt trauma to the chest or abdomen, suspect the development of shock. Also suspect the rapid development of shock in the patient who begins to display the early signs of shock (an increasing pulse rate, decreasing pulse pressure, and anxiety and restlessness) very quickly after the trauma event.

9. **Identify the need for intervention and transport of the patient with hemorrhage or shock.** **pp. 91–99**

Hemorrhage and shock are progressive pathologies that eventually become irreversible. To be effective in care, we must carefully assess our patients for the earliest of signs and intervene with rapid transport to a facility that can rapidly provide surgical intervention (to halt the internal bleeding). We also must immediately halt any external hemorrhage and provide supplemental high-flow oxygen. Intravenous fluids may be run to replace volume, but care must be used to prevent increased internal hemorrhage and hemodilution.

10. **Discuss the assessment findings and management of internal and external hemorrhage and shock.** **pp. 91–99**

Tachycardia is a compensatory cardiac action to maintain cardiac output when a reduced preload is present. A weak pulse reflects a narrowing pulse pressure and increasing peripheral vascular resistance to maintain systolic blood pressure. Cool, clammy skin is due to the redirection of blood to more critical organs than the skin. Ashen, pale skin may present due to hypoxia and peripheral vasoconstriction. Agitation, restlessness, and reduced level of consciousness occurs as the brain receives a reduced flow of oxygenated blood. The hypoxia causes the defense mechanisms of agitation and restlessness, followed by a noticeable reduction in the level of consciousness. Dull, lackluster eyes occur secondary to low perfusion and hypoxic states. Rapid, shallow respiration may occur as shock progresses, the respiratory muscles tire in the hypoxic state, and respiratory effort becomes less efficient. Dropping oxygen saturation may also provide evidence to support developing shock. As the peripheral circulation slows, the readings may drop or become erratic. Falling blood pressure heralds the progression from compensated to decompensated shock. As a late sign, it should not be used to determine the presence of shock.

External hemorrhage must be controlled by direct pressure. If direct pressure alone does not work, use elevation, pressure points or, as a last resort, the tourniquet, to stop the hemorrhage. If all sites of hemorrhage are controlled and you can rule out internal hemorrhage, provide fluid resuscitation to return the blood pressure and vital signs to normal.

Should the mechanism of injury or any early development of shock signs or symptoms suggest internal hemorrhage, or external hemorrhage cannot be controlled, transport should be expedited and care initiated immediately. Provide high-flow oxygen and ventalitory support as needed and infuse fluids to maintain the blood pressure just below 100 mmHg, ensuring it does not drop below 50 mmHg.

11. Differentiate between the administration rate and volume of IV fluid in patients with controlled versus uncontrolled hemorrhage. pp. 115–117

If hemorrhage has been controlled (as with external hemorrhage) then fluid resuscitation can be aimed at returning the blood pressure and other vital signs toward normal. However, if the hemorrhage is internal, and especially if it involves the chest, abdomen, or pelvis, great care must be exercised not to enhance the hemorrhage or excessively dilute the remaining blood. Resuscitation is generally aimed at stabilizing the blood pressure somewhere just below 100 mmHg and preventing it from dropping below 50 mmHg. To maintain these parameters, lactated Ringer's solution (preferred) or normal saline should be run rapidly through trauma or blood tubing and large-bore short catheters. Pressure infusers may be necessary as the blood pressure begins to fall below 50 mmHg. Usually prehospital care is limited to between 1 and 3 liters of crystalloid.

12. Relate pulse pressure and orthostatic vital sign changes to perfusion status. pp. 95–96, 114

Pulse pressure is the difference between the systolic and diastolic blood pressures and is responsible for the pulse. It is a relative measure of the effectiveness of cardiac output against peripheral vascular resistance. One of the early signs of shock is a decreasing pulse pressure, occurring as cardiac output begins to fall and the body increases peripheral vascular resistance in an attempt to maintain blood pressure.

Normally the body can maintain blood pressure and perfusion despite rapid changes from one position to another. However, in hypovolemia the body is already in a state of compensation so it becomes more difficult to maintain the pulse rate and blood pressure as someone moves from a supine to a seated or a standing position. If hypovolemic compensation exists, this movement will cause an increase in pulse rate and a drop in systolic blood pressure (usually by 20 points or more).

13. Define and differentiate between compensated and decompensated hemorrhagic shock. pp. 108–110

Compensated shock is a state in which the body is effectively compensating for fluid loss, or other shock-inducing pathology, and is able to maintain blood pressure and critical organ perfusion. If the original problem is not corrected or reversed, compensated shock may progress to decompensated shock.

Decompensated shock is a state in which the cardiovascular system cannot maintain critical circulation and begins to fail. Hypoxia affects the blood vessels and heart so they cannot maintain blood pressure and circulation.

Irreversible shock is a state of shock in which the human system is so damaged that it cannot be resuscitated. Once this stage of shock sets in the patient will die, even if resuscitation efforts restore a pulse and blood pressure.

14. Discuss the pathophysiological changes, assessment findings, and management associated with compensated and decompensated shock. pp. 108–110, 112–120

As the body experiences a stressor that induces shock, the cardiovascular system is quick to compensate. The venous system constricts to maintain a full vascular system and preload. The heart rate increases to maintain cardiac output, and the arterioles constrict, increasing peripheral vascular resistance to maintain blood pressure (the pressure of perfusion). As these actions become significant, the patient becomes anxious and slightly tachycardic, and the skin becomes cool and pale (circulation is shunted from the skin to more vital organs). With increasing blood loss, the compensation becomes more significant, and thirst, a rapid, weak pulse, and restlessness become apparent. These signs become more apparent as greater compensation is required to maintain the blood pressure. When the body reaches the limits of its compensation and it can no longer maintain the blood pressure, BP drops precipitously, circulation all but stops, and the patient moves very quickly into irreversible shock.

Care for the shock patient includes high-flow oxygen, hemorrhage control, and fluid resuscitation to maintain vital signs when hemorrhage is controlled, with a stable blood pressure just below 100 mmHg (88 mmHg may be optimal with continuing hemmorrhage), or use aggressive fluid resuscitation if the blood pressure drops below 50 mmHg.

15. Identify the need for intervention and transport of patients with compensated and decompensated shock. pp. 112–115

The body's ability to compensate for shock is limited. While it can maintain blood pressure, the compensation is not without cost. As the arterioles constrict, they deny blood flow to some organs and themselves use energy and tire. The venous vessels tire as they constrict to reduce the volume of the vascular system. If compensation is significant or prolonged, the body may move into decompensation, especially if the hemorrhage is not controlled. Most serious internal hemorrhage can only be halted with surgical intervention, most commonly at a trauma center. In the time between our recognition of shock and arrival at the trauma center, we can help the body with its compensation by providing oxygen and fluid resuscitation.

16. Differentiate among normotensive, hypotensive, or profoundly hypotensive patients. pp. 112–115

A normotensive patient is one who has a systolic blood pressure of at least 100 mmHg. Hypotension is the patient with a blood pressure of less than 100 mmHg, while a blood pressure of less than 50 mmHg is considered profound hypotension. However, these figures apply to the young healthy adult and must be adjusted to the norms for the patient you are treating. (For example, a small young female may normally have a blood pressure below 100 mmHg and may not need fluid resuscitation.)

17. Describe the differences in administration of intravenous fluid in normotensive, hypotensive, or profoundly hypotensive patients. pp. 115–117

Administration of intravenous fluids in the normotensive patient without hypovolemia permits the rapid administration of medications and may be indicated when hypovolemia is anticipated (the burn patient). In the patient who is in compensated shock and maintains a relatively normal systolic blood pressure, fluid resuscitation is indicated if hemorrhage is controlled. If the hemorrhage is internal and cannot be controlled in the field, aggressive fluid resuscitation may lead to increased internal hemorrhage and hemodilution making perfusion and clotting less effective. Generally, the administration of intravenous fluids in the normotensive patient is limited.

In the patient who is hypotensive (BP <100 mmHg), intravenous fluids are administered to maintain, not increase, the blood pressure. Here again aggressive fluid resuscitation would dilute the blood and decrease the effectiveness of perfusion and clotting. An increase in blood pressure would also likely break apart clots that are reducing the internal hemorrhage.

In the patient who is profoundly hypotensive (absent pulses and you are unable to determine a blood pressure, or it is < 50 mmHg), aggressive fluid resuscitation is indicated. Here the consequences of severe hypoperfusion outweigh the risks of further hemorrhage.

18. Discuss the physiologic changes associated with application and inflation of the pneumatic anti-shock garment (PASG). pp. 117–120

The pneumatic anti-shock garment (PASG) is an air bladder that circumferentially applies pressure to the lower extremities and abdomen. In theory, it compresses the venous blood vessels, returning some blood to the critical circulation, and compresses the arteries, increasing peripheral vascular resistance. These actions increase circulating blood volume and blood pressure, which should help the patient in shock. However, in some cases of shock, this may increase the rate of internal hemorrhage and may disrupt the clotting mechanisms that are restricting blood loss associated with internal injury.

19. **Discuss the indications and contraindications for the application and inflation of the PASG.** pp. 117–120

The PASG is indicated for any patient who displays internal or external hemorrhage in the lower abdomen, pelvis, or lower extremities. It is recommended for the stabilization of any pelvic fracture and may be helpful with bilateral femoral fractures with the signs and symptoms of shock.

The PASG should not be used in the patient who is experiencing pulmonary edema or has a head or penetrating chest injury. It should be used with caution on any patient who is experiencing dyspnea as it may increase intra-abdominal pressure and restrict the movement of the diaphragm. The abdominal section should not be employed if the patient is in the third trimester of pregnancy, has an abdominal evisceration, or an impaled object in the abdomen.

Prior to application of the PASG, the patient's blood pressure, pulse rate and strength, and level of consciousness should be assessed and recorded. The abdomen, lower back, and lower extremities should be visualized to ensure that no sharp debris that could harm either the patient or the garment is present.

20. **Given several preprogrammed and moulaged hemorrhage and shock patients, provide the appropriate scene size-up, initial assessment, rapid trauma assessment or focused history and physical examination, detailed physical examination, appropriate care and transport, and ongoing assessments.** pp. 78–120

During your training as an EMT-Paramedic you will participate in many classroom practice sessions involving simulated patients. You will also spend some time in the emergency departments of local hospitals as well as in advanced-level ambulances gaining clinical experience. During these times, use your knowledge of hemorrhage and shock to help you assess and care for the simulated or real patients you attend.

CASE STUDY REVIEW

Reread the case study on pages 77 and 78 in Paramedic Care: Trauma Emergencies *before reading the discussion below.*

This case study presents an example of aggressive and appropriate care for a patient who, by mechanism of injury alone, is suspected of advancing into shock. It highlights both the elements of shock assessment and care.

Arriving on the scene, Dave is presented with a situation that presents with no noticeable hazards and one patient with a mechanism of injury that indicates the potential for serious internal bleeding. The overturned bulldozer trapped the patient's legs and pelvis and may have fractured the pelvis and femurs. These injuries are frequently associated with severe internal blood loss and shock.

Dave suspects, as the vehicle is lifted off Ken, internal bleeding will occur more rapidly. In preparation, he ensures good oxygenation and assesses the visible portion of the patient. He gathers a baseline set of vital signs (all of which indicate that the patient is not yet in decompensated shock), including a pulse oximeter reading. He starts two IV lines using normal saline, one infusing wide open. He places pressure infusers over the bags, just in case they are needed. The PASG is set out on the long spine board so the patient can be moved in one step to the board and immediately have the PASG applied. Dave and his fellow rescuers converse with Ken not only to calm and reassure him, but also to maintain a continuous assessment of Ken's level of consciousness and determine a patient history. Dave requests air medical service for this patient as it may reduce the patient transport time, but since they do not arrive on scene when Ken is ready for transport, they move him by ground to the hospital. If it would save time, they might consider an intercept at a predesignated landing zone but must assure that the intercept results in a time savings.

As the bulldozer is removed, Ken is quickly assessed and then moved to the awaiting spine board. The pelvic, femoral, and tibial fractures suggest shock will develop quickly, so the PASG is inflated immediately, not only to stabilize the fractured pelvis and femurs but to tamponade the internal hemorrhage expected with these injuries. Both IVs are run wide open, and the patient is prepared for rapid transport.

Normally, fellow care providers would slow the IVs en route to the hospital; however, Ken is becoming restless, his pulse rate is increasing, and the oximetry reading is dropping. These signs herald the progression of shock and require continued aggressive care. The hospital is updated on the patient's condition so they can be ready with O-negative blood. Whole blood or packed red cells are required because the replacement of blood lost through hemorrhage with crystalloid dilutes the number of red blood cells and clotting factors available.

The hospital personnel are ready and waiting for the patient as the ambulance backs into the emergency department bay. The blood is hung and connected, and infusion is begun. The trauma surgeon makes his quick assessment, and the patient is en route to surgery in minutes.

If any one of a number of critical steps in the care of this patient had not been completed, this patient probably would not have survived the trip to the hospital. Dave moved quickly and decisively, performing the skills that stabilized his patient, yet omitting care that would have been provided had the patient not been critical. The paramedic must, through experience, be quickly able to distinguish the patient who needs rapid transport and aggressive care from the patient who will best benefit from meticulous care at the scene and during transport.

CONTENT SELF-EVALUATION

MULTIPLE CHOICE

_____ 1. Which of the following most specifically slows the heart rate?
   A. the autonomic nervous system
   B. the sympathetic nervous system
   C. the parasympathetic nervous system
   D. the somatic nervous system
   E. none of the above

_____ 2. Which of the following affects the stroke volume of the heart?
   A. preload
   B. afterload
   C. cardiac contractility
   D. ventricular filling
   E. all of the above

_____ 3. The principle that accounts for a greater force of cardiac contraction when the heart is forcefully filled with blood and the myocardium is stretched is called the:
   A. cardiac contractile force.
   B. Frank-Starling mechanism.
   C. Hering-Breuer reflex.
   D. intrinsic elasticity.
   E. Boyle's law.

_____ 4. The normal cardiac output is about:
   A. 4 liters.
   B. 5 liters.
   C. 8 liters.
   D. 10 liters.
   E. 12 liters.

_____ 5. The layer of the blood vessels that provides their smooth interior wall is the:
   A. tunica adventitia.
   B. tunica media.
   C. tunica intima.
   D. the escarpment.
   E. none of the above

_____ 6. Approximately what volume of blood is contained within the venous system?
   A. 13 percent
   B. 7 percent
   C. 64 percent
   D. 23 percent
   E. 45 percent

_____ 7. Venous constriction is able to return about what volume of blood to the active circulation?
  A. 500 mL
  B. 1,000 mL
  C. 2,000 mL
  D. 2,500 mL
  E. 3,000 mL

_____ 8. The percentage of the blood that consists of red blood cells is referred to as:
  A. its type.
  B. viscosity.
  C. the erythrocytic count.
  D. the hematocrit.
  E. none of the above

_____ 9. The blood cells responsible to help kill invading pathogens are the:
  A. erythrocytes.
  B. platelets.
  C. lymphocytes.
  D. red blood cells.
  E. both A and D

_____ 10. Which of the following types of hemorrhage is characterized by bright red blood?
  A. capillary bleeding
  B. venous bleeding
  C. arterial bleeding
  D. both A and C
  E. both A and B

_____ 11. Which of the following types of hemorrhage is characterized by dark red blood?
  A. capillary bleeding
  B. venous bleeding
  C. arterial bleeding
  D. both A and C
  E. none of the above

_____ 12. Which of the following is NOT a stage in the clotting process?
  A. intrinsic phase
  B. vascular phase
  C. platelet phase
  D. coagulation phase
  E. All of the above are phases in the clotting process.

_____ 13. Which of the following represents the phase of clotting where blood cells are trapped in fibrin strands?
  A. intrinsic phase
  B. vascular phase
  C. platelet phase
  D. coagulation phase
  E. marrow phase

_____ 14. The clotting process normally takes about what length of time?
  A. 1 to 2 minutes
  B. 3 to 4 minutes
  C. 4 to 6 minutes
  D. 7 to 10 minutes
  E. 10 to 12 minutes

_____ 15. Cleanly and transversely cut blood vessels tend to bleed very heavily.
  A. True
  B. False

_____ 16. Which of the following is likely to adversely affect the clotting process?
  A. aggressive fluid resuscitation
  B. hypothermia
  C. movement at the site of injury
  D. drugs such as aspirin
  E. all of the above

_____ 17. Bleeding from capillary or venous wounds is easy to halt because the pressure driving the hemorrhage is limited.
  A. True
  B. False

_____ 18. Fractures of the femur can account for a blood loss:
  A. from 500 to 750 mL.
  B. up to 1,500 mL.
  C. in excess of 2,000 mL.
  D. less than 500 mL.
  E. in excess of 2,500 mL.

_____ 19. The intravascular fluid accounts for what percentage of the total body water?
   A. 7 percent   D. 45 percent
   B. 15 percent   E. 75 percent
   C. 35 percent

_____ 20. In which stage of hemorrhage does the patient first display thirst?
   A. the first stage   D. the fourth stage
   B. the second stage   E. none of the above
   C. the third stage

_____ 21. In which stage of hemorrhage does the patient first display air-hunger?
   A. the first stage   D. the fourth stage
   B. the second stage   E. none of the above
   C. the third stage

_____ 22. Which of the following react differently to blood loss than the normal, healthy adult?
   A. pregnant women   D. children
   B. athletes   E. all of the above
   C. the elderly

_____ 23. The late pregnancy female is likely to have a blood volume:
   A. much less than normal.
   B. slightly less than normal.
   C. slightly greater than normal.
   D. much greater than normal.
   E. that is normal and does not change with pregnancy.

_____ 24. Obese patients are likely to have a blood volume:
   A. much less than normal.   D. much greater than normal.
   B. slightly less than normal.   E. none of the above
   C. slightly greater than normal.

_____ 25. The risk of transmitting disease to your trauma patient is probably much greater than the risk of obtaining a disease from him.
   A. True
   B. False

_____ 26. The sooner the signs and symptoms of shock appear in your patient, the greater the hemorrhage rate and the likelihood that the patient will move into the later stages of shock.
   A. True
   B. False

_____ 27. Fractures of the pelvis can account for a blood loss:
   A. from 500 to 750 mL.
   B. up to 1,500 mL.
   C. in excess of 2,000 mL.
   D. up to 500 mL.
   E. of none because the pelvis does not bleed.

_____ 28. A black, tarry stool is called:
   A. hemoptysis.   D. hematochezia.
   B. melena.   E. ebony stool.
   C. hematuria.

_____ 29. A positive tilt test demonstrating orthostatic hypotension is positive when:
   A. the blood pressure rises by at least 20 mmHg.
   B. the blood pressure falls by at least 20 mmHg.
   C. the pulse rate rises by at least 20 beats per minute.
   D. the pulse rate falls by at least 20 beats per minute.
   E. both B and C

_____ 30. For the patient in compensated shock, you should perform an ongoing assessment:
- A. every five minutes.
- B. every fifteen minutes.
- C. after every major intervention.
- D. after noting any change in signs or symptoms.
- E. all except B

_____ 31. Which of the following is a technique used to help control hemorrhage?
- A. direct pressure
- B. elevation
- C. pressure points
- D. limb splinting
- E. all of the above

_____ 32. When applying a tourniquet, you should inflate the cuff:
- A. until the bleeding slows.
- B. to the diastolic blood pressure.
- C. to the systolic blood pressure.
- D. to 30 mmHg above the systolic blood pressure.
- E. none of the above

_____ 33. Which of the following is NOT a pulse pressure point?
- A. the brachial artery
- B. the carotid artery
- C. the femoral artery
- D. the popliteal artery
- E. the radial artery

_____ 34. The aerobic component of the cell's utilization of glucose to obtain energy is called:
- A. Kreb's cycle.
- B. glycolysis.
- C. glycogenolysis.
- D. the pyruvic acid cycle.
- E. glyco cycle.

_____ 35. Under normal conditions, the blood passing the alveoli will be oxygenated to what percentage?
- A. 65 to 70
- B. 75 to 85
- C. 90 to 95
- D. 97 to 100
- E. less than 65

_____ 36. The diastolic blood pressure reflects the:
- A. strength of cardiac output.
- B. volume of cardiac output.
- C. state of peripheral vascular resistance.
- D. state of arteriole constriction.
- E. both C and D

_____ 37. Most tissues of the body can survive and perform well with blood flowing through them from 5 to 20 percent of the time.
- A. True
- B. False

_____ 38. Blood fills the vascular space EXCEPT in shock states.
- A. True
- B. False

_____ 39. Which of the following is a result of parasympathetic nervous system stimulation?
- A. decreased heart rate
- B. decreased peripheral vascular resistance
- C. decreased blood pressure
- D. decreased respiratory rate
- E. all of the above

_____ 40. Which of the following is a catecholamine?
- A. antidiuretic hormone
- B. angiotensin II
- C. aldosterone
- D. epinephrine
- E. erythropoietin

_____ 41. Which of the following is a hormone that releases steroids that, in turn, cause increased production of glucose and reduce the body's inflammatory response?
A. glucagon
B. insulin
C. norepinephrine
D. adrenocorticotropic hormone
E. none of the above

_____ 42. Erythropoietin can increase the production of erythrocytes by a factor of:
A. 2.
B. 5.
C. 10.
D. 20.
E. 25.

_____ 43. The column of coagulated erythrocytes caused by capillary stagnation is called:
A. ischemia.
B. rouleaux.
C. capillary washout.
D. hydrostatic reflux.
E. compensated reflux.

_____ 44. Which list places the stages of shock in the order of their occurrence.
A. irreversible, decompensated, compensated
B. compensated, decompensated, irreversible
C. compensated, irreversible, decompensated
D. decompensated, irreversible, compensated
E. decompensated, compensated, irreversible

_____ 45. Which stage of shock ends with a precipitous drop in blood pressure?
A. compensatory
B. decompensatory
C. irreversible
D. hypovolemic
E. none of the above

_____ 46. Which of the following does NOT occur during the compensated stage of shock?
A. increasing pulse rate
B. decreasing pulse strength
C. decreasing systolic blood pressure
D. skin becomes cool and clammy
E. the patient experiences thirst and weakness

_____ 47. Once the patient becomes profoundly unconscious and loses his vital signs, he moves into irreversible shock.
A. True
B. False

_____ 48. All of the following can cause hypovolemic shock EXCEPT:
A. bowel obstruction.
B. pancreatitis.
C. cardiac dysrhythmias.
D. ascites.
E. peritonitis.

_____ 49. Under which of the following shock types would anaphylactic shock fall?
A. hypovolemic
B. distributive
C. obstructive
D. cardiogenic
E. respiratory

_____ 50. Under which of the following shock types would tension pneumothorax fall?
A. hypovolemic
B. distributive
C. obstructive
D. cardiogenic
E. respiratory

_____ 51. Which of the following suggests shock?
A. a pulse rate above 100 in the adult
B. a pulse rate above 140 in the school-age child
C. a pulse rate above 160 in the preschooler
D. a pulse rate above 180 in the infant
E. all of the above

_____ 52. When using a pulse oximeter, you should use oxygen and ventilation to keep the reading above which oxygen saturation value?
  A. 45 percent
  B. 80 percent
  C. 85 percent
  D. 95 percent
  E. 99 percent

_____ 53. In the normotensive patient the jugular veins should be full when the patient is in the supine position.
  A. True
  B. False

_____ 54. During assessment you note that the patient's lower extremities and lower abdomen are warm and pink while the upper extremities, thorax, and upper abdomen are cool and clammy. This presentation is consistent with which type of shock?
  A. hypovolemic
  B. neurogenic
  C. obstructive
  D. cardiogenic
  E. respiratory

_____ 55. Which of the following may be an indication to employ overdrive respiration?
  A. severe rib fractures
  B. flail chest
  C. diaphragmatic respirations
  D. head injury
  E. all of the above

_____ 56. Which of these fluid replacement choices would be most desirable for the patient who is losing blood through internal bleeding?
  A. packed red blood cells
  B. fresh frozen plasma
  C. whole blood
  D. colloids
  E. crystalloids

_____ 57. Most of the solutions used in prehospital care for infusion are:
  A. hypotonic colloids.
  B. isotonic colloids.
  C. hypertonic colloids.
  D. hypotonic crystalloids.
  E. isotonic crystalloids.

_____ 58. Which of the following characteristics of a catheter will ensure that fluids run rapidly through it?
  A. short length, small lumen
  B. short length, large lumen
  C. long length, small lumen
  D. long length, large lumen
  E. large lumen and either long or short length

_____ 59. In the patient that has internal bleeding and hypovolemia, the objective blood pressure to maintain by PASG and fluid infusions is:
  A. 120 mmHg.
  B. 100 mmHg.
  C. 50 mmHg.
  D. below 50 mmHg.
  E. at a steady level.

_____ 60. The PASG may return what volume of blood to the central circulation?
  A. 250 mL
  B. 500 mL
  C. 750 mL
  D. 1,000 mL
  E. none at all

SPECIAL PROJECTS

Scenario-Based Problem Solving

You are caring for a victim of a single stab wound to the left upper quadrant. He is a 36-year-old male who is conscious, alert, and oriented, though somewhat agitated. His initial vitals are BP: 120/90, pulse: 110 and weak, respirations 20 with clear breath sounds, and his skin is somewhat cool and moist.

1. What organs might be injured by this mechanism?

   _____

   _____

2. Why is the patient somewhat agitated?

   _____

   _____

   _____

3. If this patient's normal BP is 120/80, what would explain the increased diastolic blood pressure?

   _____

   _____

4. What is the relationship between the increased diastolic blood pressure and the weak pulse?

   _____

   _____

   _____

5. Why is the skin somewhat cool and clammy?

   _____

   _____

   _____

Drip Math Worksheet 1

Formulas

Rate = Volume/Time   mL/min = gtts per min/gtts per mL

Volume = Rate × Time   gtts/min = mL per min × gtts per mL

Time = Volume/Rate   mL = gtts/gtts per mL

Please complete the following drug and drip math problems:

1. Upon arriving at the emergency department the physician asks how much fluid you infused into your trauma patient. Your on-scene and transport time was 35 minutes, and you ran normal saline at a rate of 120 gtts/minute through a 10 gtts/mL administration set. What would you report?

2. Protocol calls for a drug to be hung and administered by drip at 45 gtts per minute based upon a 60 gtts/mL administration set. You find that the set you have administers 45 gtts/mL. How many drops per second should you set your chamber for?

3. The transferring physician requests that you infuse 100 mL of a drug during your transport. Anticipated transport time is 1 hour and 55 minutes. At what rate would you set a 60 gtts/mL administration set?

4. You are allowed to administer a drug by IV drip at a rate of between 45 and 100 mL per hour. What drip rate range can you use with a

   60 gtts/mL set?

   45 gtts/mL set?

   10 gtts/mL set?

5. After a call, you can't remember at what rate you ran a fluid. You do know that 350 mL are left in the 500 mL bag and that the IV was running for 1 hour and 5 minutes. What would you record?

CHAPTER 5
✳
Soft-Tissue Trauma

Review of Chapter Objectives

After reading this chapter, you should be able to:

1. Describe the incidence, morbidity, and mortality of soft-tissue injures.   pp. 125–126

Soft tissue injuries are by far the most prevalent type of injuries to occur, accounting for over 10 million visits to the emergency department yearly. Any mechanism of injury affecting the human system must first penetrate the skin and then the soft tissues to injure any organ. However, soft-tissue injuries rarely by themselves threaten life. Open injuries to the skin may permit pathogens to enter and infection to develop, and significant wounds may cause cosmetic and, to some degree, functional disruption of the skin. Injuries to the skin may also permit significant hemorrhage.

2. Describe the anatomy and physiology of the integumentary system, including:

The integumentary system is the largest body organ, accounting for about 16 percent of weight. It provides the outer barrier for the body and protects it against environmental extremes, fluid loss, and pathogen invasion. The three-layer structure consists of:

a. Epidermis   pp. 126–127
The epidermis is the most superficial layer of the skin and consists of numerous layers of dead or dying cells. The epidermis provides a flexible covering for the skin and a barrier to fluid loss, absorption, and the entrance of pathogens.

b. Dermis   p. 127
The dermis is the true skin. It is made up of connective tissue and houses the sensory nerve endings, many of the specialized skin cells that produce sweat, oil, etc., and the upper-level capillary beds that allow for the conduction of heat to the body's surface.

c. Subcutaneous tissue   pp. 127–128
The subcutaneous layer, although not a true part of the skin, works in concert with the skin to insulate the body from heat loss and the effects of trauma. It consists of connective and adipose (fatty) tissues.

3. Identify the skin tension lines of the body.   pp. 129–130

The skin is a flexible cover for the body and as such is firmly connected to some parts of the anatomy while at other locations it is somewhat mobile. Its elasticity permits a wide range of motion by the musculoskeletal system while maintaining its own integrity. This elasticity creates tension along lines (called skin tension lines) that will cause a wound to gape or remain somewhat closed based upon its orientation to the skin tension lines. Please see the illustration (Figure 5-3) on page 130 of the textbook.

4. Predict soft-tissue injuries based on mechanism of injury. pp. 130–136, 149–152

Blunt trauma is most likely to produce closed soft-tissue injury such as a contusion or hematoma, especially when the tissue is trapped between the force and skeletal structures like the ribs or skull. Crush injury occurs as the soft tissue is trapped in machinery or under a very heavy object. Penetrating trauma occurs as an object passes through the soft tissues, introducing pathogens to the body's interior and creating the risk of infection. Penetrating injury is likely to produce lacerations, incisions, and punctures as well as internal hemorrhage. Shear and tearing injuries may result in avulsions or amputation.

5. Discuss blunt and penetrating trauma. pp. 130–136

Blunt trauma is a kinetic force spread out over a relatively large surface area and directed at the body. It is most likely to induce injuries that do not break the skin, including contusions, and internal hemorrhage between the fascia, or hematomas. The stretching forces caused by blunt trauma, if significant enough, may cause a tear in the skin (laceration) and an open wound. Compression-type injuries can cause crushing wounds where the tissues and blood vessels and nerves are crushed, stretched, and torn.

Penetrating trauma, depending upon its exact mechanism, may cause a laceration (a jagged cut), an incision (a very precise or surgical cut), or a puncture (a deep wound with an opening that closes). Tearing or shear forces may cause an avulsion (a tearing away of skin), or an amputation (a complete severance or tearing away of a digit or limb). Scraping forces may abrade away the upper layers of skin and produce an abrasion.

6. Discuss the pathophysiology of soft-tissue injuries. pp. 130–146

Soft-tissue injuries either damage blood vessels and the structure of the soft tissue (blunt trauma) or open the envelope of the skin (penetrating trauma) and may permit pathogens to enter and blood to escape. Blunt trauma includes contusions, hematomas, and crush injuries. Penetrating trauma includes abrasions, lacerations, incisions, punctures, impaled objects, avulsions and amputations. Soft-tissue wounds may also present with hemorrhage, either capillary (oozing), venous (flowing), or arterial (spurting). The hemorrhage may be external or internal. Once injured, the soft tissue has the ability to heal itself through hemostasis, inflammation, epithelialization, neovascularization, and collagen synthesis. It also is able, through the recruitment of blood cells (phagocytes), to combat invading pathogens and prevent or combat infection. Infection risk is increased with pre-existing diseases like COPD or with diseases that compromise the immune system like HIV infection and AIDS. Use of medications like the NSAIDs also affects infection risk. The contamination introduced into the wound, the wound site (distal extremities), and the nature of the wound (puncture, crush, and avulsion) also have an impact on the risk of infection.

7. Differentiate among the following types of soft-tissue injuries:

a. Closed pp. 130–133

i. Contusion
A contusion is a closed wound caused by blunt trauma that damages small blood vessels. The blood vessels leak, and the affected area becomes edematous. The contusion is characterized by swelling, pain, and, later on, discoloration. Since the wound is closed, the danger of infection is remote.

ii. Hematoma
The hematoma is a blunt soft-tissue injury in which blood vessels (larger than capillaries) are damaged and leak into the fascia, causing a pocket of blood. Large hematomas may accumulate up to 500 mL of blood.

iii. Crush injuries
Crush injuries occur as the soft tissues are trapped between a compressing force and an unyeilding object and extensive injury occurs. The injury disrupts blood vessels, nerves,

muscle, connective tissue, bone, and possibly internal organs. Such an injury often provides a challenge to management because there is often serious bleeding from numerous sources and the nature of the wound makes the bleeding hard to control. Open crush injuries are frequently associated with severe infection.

b. Open pp. 133–136

i. Abrasions
An abrasion is a scraping away of the upper layers of the skin. It will normally present with capillary bleeding, and since the wound is open and may involve an extended surface, it can be associated with infection.

ii. Lacerations
Laceration is the most common open wound. It is a tear into the layers of the skin and, sometimes, deeper. A laceration can involve blood vessels, muscles, connective tissue, and other underlying structures. Since it is an open wound, it carries with it the danger of infection and external hemorrhage.

iii. Incisions
The incision is a very smooth laceration made by a surgical or other sharp instrument. It is otherwise a laceration.

iv. Avulsions
An avulsion is a partial tearing away of the skin and soft tissues. It is commonly associated with blunt skull trauma, animal bites, or machinery accidents. The degloving injury is a form of avulsion.

v. Impaled objects
An impaled object is any object that enters and then is lodged within the soft or other tissue. While its entry poses an infection risk, removing the object risks increased hemorrhage because the impaled object may be tamponading blood loss. Removal may also cause further harm if the object is irregular in shape.

vi. Amputations
An amputation is the partial or complete severance of a body part. The injury usually results in the complete loss of the limb distal to the site of severance; however, the severed limb can sometimes be successfully reattached or its tissue may be used for grafting to extend the length and usefulness of the remaining limb.

vii. Punctures
Punctures are penetrating wounds into the skin where the nature of the wound (deep and narrow) encourages closure. Pathogens driven into the wound by the mechanism find a hypoxic environment and may thrive in the injured tissue, resulting in serious infection.

8. Discuss the assessment and management of open and closed soft-tissue injuries. pp. 149–168

In the prehospital setting, the assessment of soft-tissue injuries is straightforward. In fact, soft-tissue injuries may be the only physical indications of serious internal injuries underneath. The assessment of these internal injuries is only complicated because the discoloration normally associated with them takes a few hours to develop. Examine the skin for any deformity, discoloration, or variation in temperature. Visualize any noted wound and determine its nature and extent. Be able to describe it (as it will be covered by a dressing and bandaging) to the attending physician upon your arrival at the emergency department.

The management of a soft-tissue wound is simply accomplished by meeting three objectives: immobilizing the wound site, keeping the wound clean (as sterile as possible), and controlling any hemorrhage. Immobilization will assist the clotting and healing processes. Keeping the wound sterile will reduce the bacterial load and reduce the risk and severity of infection. Controlling the hemorrhage with the use of direct pressure will limit blood loss and speed the repair cycle. In most circumstances, direct pressure effectively controls hemorrhage. Occasionally both direct pressure and elevation of the limb may be necessary. In severe cases of hemorrhage, the use of pressure points will be needed in addition to direct pressure and elevation. In extreme cases, such as severe crush injury, a tourniquet may be needed.

9. Discuss the incidence, morbidity, and mortality of crush injuries. 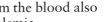 pp. 132–133, 163–166

Crush injury is an infrequent mechanism that often results in severe soft tissue damage. The extensive nature of the injury predisposes it to infection, which can be severe. Entrapment of a limb or body region may lead to crush syndrome in which a prolonged lack of circulation leads to the breakdown of muscle tissues and to rhabdomyolysis. Reperfusion of the affected region then transports myoglobin to the kidneys, threatening renal failure, and potassium to the heart, causing dysrhythmias or sudden death.

10. Define the following injuries:

a. Crush injury pp. 132–133, 144–145

Crush injury occurs when a part of the body is trapped between a force and an object resisting it. Such injuries may occur as a limb is trapped in machinery, under a car as a jack releases, or in a building collapse. The injury disrupts the soft, connective, vascular, and nervous tissue and may injure internal organs.

b. Crush syndrome pp. 145, 163–165

Crush syndrome occurs as a body part is trapped for more than four hours. The reduced or absent circulation within the trapped part does not permit the supply of oxygen and nutrients nor does it allow removal of carbon dioxide and waste products. The tissues become hypoxic and acidotic, and waste products accumulate. Upon release of the entrapping pressure, these toxins are returned to the central circulation with very severe effects. Fluid from the blood also flows into the injured tissue, resulting in a significant contribution to hypovolemia.

c. Compartment syndrome pp. 143, 165–166

Compartment syndrome occurs as edema increases the pressure within a fascial compartment of the body. The pressure restricts venous flow from the extremity, capillary flow through the affected portion of the limb, and arterial return to the central circulation. The result of untreated compartment syndrome is often loss of some of the muscle mass and possibly the shortening of the muscle mass.

11. Discuss the mechanisms of injury, assessment findings, and management of crush injuries. pp. 144–145, 163–166

Crush injuries occur as soft tissues are trapped between two forces. The result is damage to the soft tissues, blood vessels, nerves, muscles, and bones. The limb or region that is crushed may appear normal or may be quite disfigured. Distal sensation and circulation may be disrupted, and the wound may not bleed at all or hemorrhage severely with no distinct site of hemorrhage. The limb may also feel hard and "boardlike" as hypoxia and acidosis cause the muscles to contract. Management of the crush injury follows routine soft-tissue injury care with special emphasis on hemorrhage control (use of a tourniquet may be necessary), keeping the wound clean (as the crush injury is at increased risk for infection), and elevating the limb (to enhance venous return and distal circulation).

12. Discuss the effects of reperfusion and rhabdomyolysis on the body. pp. 145, 163–166

As a limb or other body region is compressed for more than 4 hours, the lack of circulation causes a destruction of muscle tissue (rhabdomyolysis). This destruction releases a protein, myoglobin, and phosphate, potassium, and lactic and uric acids. When compression is released, reperfusion returns these toxins to the central circulation. Myoglobin clogs the tubules of the kidneys, especially when the patient is in hypovolemic shock. This may result in renal failure and, ultimately, death. More immediate, however, is the effect of the release of electrolytes on the heart. That release may result in dysrhythmias or sudden death. Other effects of reperfusion include calcification of the vasculature or of nervous tissue and increased cellular and systemic acidosis as restored circulation permits the production of uric acid.

13. **Discuss the pathophysiology, assessment, and care of hemorrhage associated with soft-tissue injuries, including:**

a. **Capillary bleeding**   p. 154

Capillary bleeding oozes from the wound and usually continues for a few minutes as the capillaries do not have the musculature to constrict as do the arteries and veins. The hemorrhage is usually minimal and can easily be controlled with the application of a dressing and minimal pressure.

b. **Venous bleeding**   p. 154

Venous hemorrhage may be extensive as the volume flowing through the vessels is equivalent to the amount flowing through arteries though the pressure of flow is much less. Venous hemorrhage is limited as the injured vessel constricts and clotting mechanisms are usually effective. Simple direct pressure will easily stop most venous hemorrhage.

c. **Arterial bleeding**   pp. 154–156

Arterial hemorrhage is powered by the blood pressure and, if the wound is open, may spurt bright red blood. The musculature of the arterial vessels will constrict to limit hemorrhage, but bleeding will likely still be heavy. Direct pressure must be applied to the bleeding site to effectively control it; in some cases, use of elevation and pressure points will be necessary.

Basically, hemorrhage can be controlled by employing direct pressure, elevation, proximal arterial pressure, and, if all else fails, a tourniquet.

Direct pressure is a very effective first-line technique for the control of hemorrhage. Since hemorrhage is powered by blood pressure, digital pressure at the site of blood loss should easily stop most blood loss.

Elevation can be used to complement direct pressure. Elevating an extremity decreases the blood pressure to the limb, and the hemorrhage may be easier to control. Use elevation only for wounds on otherwise uninjured limbs, and only after direct pressure alone has proved ineffective.

Use of a pressure point is an adjunct to both direct pressure and elevation. A proximal artery is located and compressed, reducing the pressure of the hemorrhage. Use of pressure points can be very helpful in the crush wound where the exact location of blood loss is difficult to locate.

The tourniquet is the last technique to be used in attempts to control hemorrhage. A limb is circumferentially compressed above the systolic pressure under a wide band, such as a blood pressure cuff. If a lower pressure is used, the wound will bleed more severely. The tourniquet carries with it the additional hazard of permitting toxins to accumulate in the unoxygenated limb. These toxins endanger the future use of the limb and, when released into the central circulation, the patient's life.

14. **Describe and identify the indications for and application of the following dressings and bandages:**   pp. 146–148

a. **Sterile/nonsterile dressing**

Sterile dressings are used for wound care as it is important to reduce the amount of contamination at a wound site to reduce the risk of infection.

b. **Occlusive/nonocclusive dressing**

Most dressings are nonocclusive, which means they permit both blood and air to travel through them in at least a limited way. Occlusive dressings do not permit the flow of either fluid or air and are useful in sealing a chest or neck wound to prevent the aspiration of air or covering a moist dressing on an abdominal evisceration to prevent its drying.

c. **Adherent/nonadherent dressing**

Adherent dressings support the clotting mechanisms; however, as they are removed they will dislodge the forming clots. Most dressings are specially treated to be nonadherent to prevent reinjury when they are removed from a wound.

d. **Absorbent/nonabsorbent dressing**

Most dressings used to treat wounds are absorbent, and they will soak up blood and other fluids. Nonabsorbent dressings absorb little or no fluid and are used to seal wound sites when a barrier to leaking is desired, for example, with the clear membranes that are used to cover venipuncture sites.

e. Wet/dry dressing
Wet dressings may provide a medium for the movement of infectious agents and are not frequently used in prehospital care. They may be used for abdominal eviscerations and burns.

f. Self-adherent roller bandage
The self-adherent roller bandage is soft, gauze-like material that molds to the contours of the body and is effective in holding dressings in place. As its stretch is limited, it does not pose the danger of increasing the bandaging pressure with each wrap as do some other bandaging materials.

g. Gauze bandage
Gauze bandaging is a self-adherent material that does not stretch and may increase the pressure beneath the bandage with consecutive wraps or with edema and swelling from the wound.

h. Adhesive bandage
An adhesive bandage is a strong gauze, paper, or plastic material backed with an adhesive. It can effectively secure small dressings to the skin where circumferential wrapping is impractical. It is inelastic and will not accommodate edema or swelling.

i. Elastic bandage
An elastic bandage is made of fabric that stretches easily. It conforms well to body contours but will increase the pressure applied with each wrap of the bandage. These bandages are often used to help strengthen a joint or apply pressure to reduce edema but should be used with great care, if at all, in the prehospital setting.

15. Predict the possible complications of an improperly applied dressing or bandage.   pp. 146–148, 160

Improper application of a dressing may include use of the wrong dressing for the injury or the application of the right dressing in an incorrect manner. Use of a nonocclusive dressing with an open chest would may permit air to enter the thorax, increasing the severity of a pneumothorax, or use of such a dressing for a neck wound may permit air to enter the jugular vein, creating pulmonary emboli. Use of dry dressings with an abdominal evisceration may permit tissues to dry, adding additional injury, while use of wet dressings in other circumstances provides a route for infection of wounds. Adherent dressings may facilitate natural clotting but may dislodge clots and re-institute hemorrhage as they are removed. If a dressing is too large for the wound, it may not permit application of adequate direct pressure to arrest hemorrhage. If a dressing is too small, it may become lost in the wound and again not provide a focused direct pressure to stop hemorrhage.

Improperly applied bandaging may either be insufficient to immobilize the dressing or to protect it from catching on items during care and transport. It may be too tight, restricting edema and swelling and compressing the soft tissues beneath, which can cause reduced or absent blood flow to the distal extremity. In such a case, the bandaging acts as a venous tourniquet and may actually increase the rate of hemorrhage as it increases the venous pressure. On the other hand, a bandage that is too loose may not maintain adequate direct pressure to stop bleeding or may not hold the dressing securely to the injury site.

16. Discuss the process of wound healing, including:

a. Hemostasis   pp. 138–139
Hemostasis is the process by which the body tries to restrict or halt blood loss. It begins with the constriction of the injured blood vessel wall to reduce the rate of hemorrhage. The injured tissue of the vessel wall and the platelets become sticky. The platelets then aggregate to further occlude the lumen. Finally, the clotting cascade produces fibrin strands that trap erythrocytes and form a more durable clot to halt all but the most severe hemorrhage.

b. Inflammation p. 139

Cells damaged by trauma or invading pathogens signal the body to recruit white blood cells (phagocytes) to the injury site. These cells engulf or attack the membranes of the foreign agents. The byproducts of this action cause the mast cells to release histamine, which dilates precapillary vessels and increases capillary permeability. Fluid and oxygen flows into the region resulting in an increase in temperature and edema.

c. Epithelialization p.139

The stratum germinativum cells of the epidermis create an expanding layer of cells over the wound edges. This layer eventually joins almost unnoticeably, or, if the wound is too large, a region of collagen may show through (scar tissue).

d. Neovascularization p.140

Neovascularization occurs as the capillaries surrounding the wound extend into the new tissue and begin to provide the new tissue with circulation. These new vessels are very delicate and prone to injury and tend to bleed easily.

e. Collagen synthesis p. 140

Collagen synthesis is the building of new connective tissue (collagen) in the wound through the actions of the fibroblasts. Collagen binds the wound margins together and strengthens the healing wound. The early repair is not as good as new but by the fourth month the wound tissue is about 60 percent of the original tissue's strength.

17. Discuss the assessment and management of wound healing. pp. 137–142

Wound healing is most commonly complicated by movement of the injury site or by infection. Injuries affecting joints, other locations associated with movement, or regions with poor circulation are most prone to improper wound healing. Immobilization can help the process. Infection is a common complication of open soft-tissue injuries and results in delayed or incomplete wound healing. Wound healing is best managed by keeping the site immobilized (within reason) and keeping the site as sterile as possible, with frequent dressing changes. In some cases, wound drainage may help remove the products of pathogen breakdown and enhance the recovery and healing process.

18. Discuss the pathophysiology, assessment, and management of wound infection. pp. 140–146

Next to hemorrhage, infection is the most common complication of open soft-tissue wounds. It occurs as pathogens are introduced into the wound site and grow, usually in the damaged, warm, and hypoxic tissues. The most common infectious agents are of the Staphylococcus and Streptococcus bacterial families. It takes a few days for the bacteria to grow to the numbers necessary for the development of significant signs and symptoms. Consequently, infection is not usually seen during emergency care. The site of infection is generally swollen, reddened, and warm to the touch. A foul-smelling collection of white blood cells, dead bacteria, and cellular debris (pus) may drain from the wound, and visible red streaks (lymphangitis) may extend from the wound margins toward the trunk. The patient may complain of fever and malaise. The management of an infected wound includes keeping the wound clean, permitting it to drain, and administering antibiotics.

19. Formulate treatment priorities for patients with soft-tissue injuries in conjunction with:

a. Airway/face/neck trauma pp. 166–167

Soft-tissue injury to the face and neck generally heals well due to the more than adequate circulation in the area. However, these wounds, due to their prominence, deserve special attention because of their cosmetic implications. They also deserve special concern because of the potential danger to the airway. First, assure the airway is patent and not in danger of being obstructed from either hemorrhage or swelling. Intubate early, possibly with rapid sequence intubation, to assure the airway remains patent. In the most severe cases, cricothyrotomy (needle or surgical) may be necessary. If there are any open wounds to the neck, assure they are covered with occlusive dressings to prevent the passage of air into the jugular veins.

b. Thoracic trauma (open/closed)
p. 167

Anticipate internal chest injury associated with superficial soft-tissue injuries to the thorax and cover any significant open wounds with occlusive dressings sealed on three sides. Auscultate the chest frequently to monitor respiratory exchange and anticipate progressive chest pathologies, increasing edema, or pneumothorax. Also anticipate associated internal hemorrhage and abdominal injuries and move quickly to transport the patient to a trauma center.

c. Abdominal trauma
pp. 167–168

In cases of abdominal trauma, consider the possibility of internal injury and dress all open wounds. Anticipate internal hemorrhage and move quickly to transport the patient to a trauma center. Cover any abdominal eviscerations with moistened sterile dressings, and then cover with occlusive dressings.

20. Given several scenarios involving moulaged soft-tissue injury patients, provide the appropriate assessment and field management. pp. 149–169

During your training as an EMT-Paramedic you will participate in many classroom practice sessions involving simulated patients. You will also spend some time in the emergency departments of local hospitals as well as in advanced-level ambulances gaining clinical experience. During these times, use your knowledge of soft-tissue injuries to help you assess and care for the simulated or real patients you attend.

CASE STUDY REVIEW

Reread the case study on pages 124 and 125 in Paramedic Care: Trauma Emergencies *before reading the discussion below.*
This case study depicts a serious injury to the soft tissues and the most common causes for concern with those injuries, serious hemorrhage and underlying structure injury. It gives us the opportunity to examine the assessment and care for this common injury.

Maria and Jon respond to a patient with deep soft-tissue injury involving the upper left arm. They don gloves as a standard body substance isolation precaution but also employ goggles because the wound is bleeding heavily and may involve arterial hemorrhage and the possible danger of splashing blood. Their survey of the scene reveals no indication of violence or other hazards to themselves or their patient. They recognize no other patients and see no need for additional resources.

During their initial assessment, Maria and Jon form an initial impression of Walter and determine that he is alert, oriented, and otherwise appears healthy. Since he is easily able to articulate in full sentences, they presume his airway is clear and his breathing is adequate. They note that his skin is slightly pale and his pulse is somewhat rapid, due either to excitement and the release of adrenaline or to the early signs of hypovolemia compensation and shock. At the end of the initial assessment, the paramedic team does not consider Walter a candidate for rapid transport. However, they will watch for the early or progressing signs of shock and modify that decision at any time during the remaining assessment and care. They will be especially watchful for an increasing heart rate, a weakening pulse (dropping pulse pressure), or any signs of agitation, nervousness, or combativeness from Walter.

Maria and Jon then perform a focused assessment, looking specifically at the wound to assess its nature, to determine what hemorrhage control techniques are best and to be able to describe the wound accurately to the attending physician when they arrive at the emergency department. They also examine the distal extremity for loss of nervous control or circulation. They note some patient complaint of tingling, and Walter's inability to flex his elbow. They also check both capillary refill time and neurologic function of the injured extremity and compare them against those of the opposite extremity.

As a final assessment step, the paramedics remove the rag applied by Walter, examine the wound carefully, and then cover it with sterile dressings held firmly in place with soft roller bandaging, wrapped tightly to apply direct pressure. They suspect only venous hemorrhage from their exam of the wound and may elevate the extremity once Walter is loaded on the stretcher. This enhances venous return through the injured extremity and will help reduce any continuing blood loss.

Maria and Jon use the AMPLE mnemonic to investigate Walter's medical history and discover that he has not had a recent tetanus booster. This is an important finding, as he will need to receive a booster once at the emergency department. It is also important that they investigate any allergy to the "caine" family of drugs because Walter will likely receive some form of local anesthetic during care. It is also important to investigate any antibiotic and analgesic use.

Finally, the paramedics of Medic 151 provide serial ongoing assessments of Walter and his wound. They reassess the vital signs, Walter's level of consciousness, and the dressing and bandage to ensure that there are no signs of progressing shock or continuing hemorrhage.

CONTENT SELF-EVALUATION

MULTIPLE CHOICE

_____ 1. About what percentage of soft-tissue wounds become infected, with a significant resultant morbidity?
A. 2 percent
D. 50 percent
B. 7 percent
E. 75 percent
C. 15 percent

_____ 2. Which of the following glands secrete sweat?
A. sudoriferous glands
D. adrenal glands
B. sebaceous glands
E. none of the above
C. subcutaneous glands

_____ 3. Which of the following types of cells are found in the dermis?
A. lymphocytes
D. fibroblasts
B. macrophages
E. all of the above
C. mast cells

_____ 4. The layers of the arteries and veins proceeding in order from exterior to interior are the:
A. intima, media, adventitia.
D. adventitia, media, intima.
B. media, intima, adventitia.
E. intima, adventitia, media.
C. adventitia, intima, media.

_____ 5. The blood vessels responsible for distributing blood to the major regions and organs of the body are the:
A. arteries.
D. venules.
B. arterioles.
E. veins.
C. capillaries.

_____ 6. The blood vessels able to change their lumen size by a factor of five are the:
A. arteries.
D. venules.
B. arterioles.
E. veins.
C. capillaries.

_____ 7. The sheet of thick, fibrous material surrounding muscles is the:
A. sebum.
D. tension line.
B. fascia.
E. tunica.
C. tendon.

_____ 8. Lacerations that run parallel to skin tension lines will cause the wound to gape.
A. True
B. False

_____ 9. Which of the following types of wounds are unlikely to heal well?
A. wounds that gape
B. wound associated with static tension lines
C. wounds associated with dynamic tension lines
D. wounds perpendicular to tension lines
E. all except B

_____ 10. The type of wound characterized by erythema usually seen during the prehospital setting is the:
   A. abrasion.
   B. contusion.
   C. laceration.
   D. incision.
   E. avulsion.

_____ 11. Which of the following wounds is not considered open?
   A. laceration
   B. abrasion
   C. contusion
   D. puncture
   E. avulsion

_____ 12. Which of the following wound types is characterized as a very clean, open wound?
   A. abrasion
   B. contusion
   C. laceration
   D. incision
   E. avulsion

_____ 13. Crush injuries usually involve injury to:
   A. blood vessels.
   B. nerves.
   C. bones.
   D. internal structures.
   E. all of the above

_____ 14. Which of the following is NOT usually considered an open wound?
   A. abrasion
   B. crush injury
   C. incision
   D. degloving injury
   E. avulsion

_____ 15. The wound that poses the greatest risk for serious infection is the:
   A. puncture.
   B. laceration.
   C. contusion.
   D. incision.
   E. hematoma.

_____ 16. The injury in which the skin is pulled off a finger, hand, or extremity by farm or industrial machinery is called a(n):
   A. amputation.
   B. incision.
   C. complete laceration.
   D. degloving injury.
   E. transection.

_____ 17. Amputations that occur cleanly are likely to be associated with severe hemorrhage.
   A. True
   B. False

_____ 18. The natural tendency of the body to maintain its normal environment and function is called:
   A. anemia.
   B. homeostasis.
   C. hemostasis.
   D. coagulation.
   E. metabolism.

_____ 19. When torn or cut, the muscles in the capillaries constrict, thereby limiting hemorrhage.
   A. True
   B. False

_____ 20. The agents that recruit cells responsible for the inflammatory response are called:
   A. macrophages.
   B. lymphocytes.
   C. chemotactic factors.
   D. granulocytes.
   E. fibroblasts.

_____ 21. The cells that attack invading pathogens directly or through an antibody response are:
   A. macrophages.
   B. lymphocytes.
   C. white blood cells.
   D. granulocytes.
   E. fibroblasts.

_____ 22. The stage of the healing process in which the phagocytes and lymphocytes are most active is:
A. inflammation.
B. epithelialization.
C. neovascularization.
D. collagen synthesis.
E. none of the above

_____ 23. Regenerated skin, after about four months, is about how strong as compared to the original skin?
A. 20 percent
B. 30 percent
C. 40 percent
D. 50 percent
E. 60 percent

_____ 24. Infection usually appears how long after the initial wound?
A. 12 to 24 hours
B. 1 to 2 days
C. 2 to 3 days
D. 4 to 6 days
E. 7 to 10 days

_____ 25. Which of the following is an infection risk factor with soft-tissue wounds?
A. advancing age
B. crush injury
C. NSAIDs use
D. cat bites
E. all of the above

_____ 26. Closing wounds with staples or sutures increases the risk of infection.
A. True
B. False

_____ 27. It is common practice to provide tetanus boosters if the patient's last booster was over:
A. 1 year ago.
B. 2 years ago.
C. 3 years ago.
D. 4 years ago.
E. 5 years ago.

_____ 28. Which of the following can interfere with normal clotting?
A. aspirin
B. warfarin
C. streptokinase
D. penicillin
E. all of the above

_____ 29. The location at greatest risk for compartment syndrome is the:
A. calf.
B. thigh.
C. forearm.
D. arm.
E. ankle.

_____ 30. The excessive growth of scar tissue within the boundaries of the wound is called:
A. hypertrophic scar formation.
B. keloid scar formation.
C. anatropic scar formation.
D. residual scar formation.
E. regressive scar formation.

_____ 31. The nature of crush injury produces an injury area that is an excellent growth medium for infection.
A. True
B. False

_____ 32. A crush injury that produces crush syndrome usually requires what minimum time of entrapment?
A. 1 hour
B. 2 hours
C. 4 hours
D. 6 hours
E. 10 hours

_____ 33. Which of the following is likely with the release of entrapment in the patient suffering crush syndrome?
A. kidney failure
B. cardiac dysrhythmias
C. hypovolemia
D. abnormal vascular calcifications
E. all of the above

_____ 34. The type of dressing that prevents the movement of fluid or air through the dressing is:
   A. sterile.
   B. nonadherent.
   C. absorbent.
   D. occlusive.
   E. nonocclusive.

_____ 35. The bandages that increase pressure beneath the bandage with each consecutive wrap are:
   A. elastic bandages.
   B. self-adherent roller bandages.
   C. gauze bandages.
   D. adhesive bandages.
   E. triangular bandages.

_____ 36. Not only is the skin the first body organ to experience trauma, it is often the only one to display the signs of injury.
   A. True
   B. False

_____ 37. Which of the following are important factors to consider in the assessment and management of external hemorrhage?
   A. type of bleeding
   B. rate of hemorrhage
   C. volume of blood lost
   D. stopping further hemorrhage
   E. all of the above

_____ 38. Which of the following is one of the primary objectives of bandaging?
   A. neat appearance
   B. hemorrhage control
   C. allowing easy movement of the wound
   D. debridement
   E. aeration

_____ 39. Insufficient tourniquet pressure may increase the rate and volume of hemorrhage.
   A. True
   B. False

_____ 40. The restoration of circulation once a tourniquet is released may cause which of the following?
   A. shock
   B. hypovolemia
   C. lethal dysrhythmias
   D. renal failure
   E. all of the above

_____ 41. After bandaging a patient's severely hemorrhaging forearm wound, you notice that the limb is cool, capillary refill is slowed, and the radial pulse cannot be found. You should:
   A. apply more dressing material and increase the pressure.
   B. leave the bandage as it is.
   C. loosen the bandage.
   D. elevate the extremity and assess circulation again.
   E. remove the bandage.

_____ 42. To alleviate pain associated with soft-tissue injury, you should administer morphine sulfate:
   A. 10 mg IV.
   B. 2 mg every 5 minutes titrated to pain relief.
   C. 5 mg every 5 minutes titrated to pain relief.
   D. 10 mg every 10 minutes times 2.
   E. 20 mg every 5 minutes titrated to pain relief.

_____ 43. With a large and gaping wound to the neck, use a(n):
   A. large absorbent dressing.
   B. large nonadherent dressing.
   C. occlusive dressing.
   D. nonabsorbent dressing.
   E. triangular bandage.

_____ 44. The type of dressing recommended for blood and fluid leaking from the auditory canal is a(n):
A. nonocclusive dressing.
B. nonadherent dressing.
C. occlusive dressing.
D. gauze dressing.
E. wet dressing.

_____ 45. Which of the following is NOT a distal sign that a circumferential bandage is too tight?
A. diaphoresis
B. pallor
C. loss of pulses
D. tingling
E. swelling

_____ 46. You find a patient who has suffered a finger amputation. You should keep the amputated part:
A. warm and dry.
B. warm and moist.
C. cool and dry.
D. cool and moist.
E. packed in ice.

_____ 47. If the amputated part cannot be immediately located, wait only a few minutes at the scene as its transport with the patient is extremely important.
A. True
B. False

_____ 48. In which of the following situations is removal of an impaled object allowed or required?
A. The object obstructs the airway.
B. The object prevents performance of CPR.
C. The object is impaled in the cheek.
D. The object is impaled in the chest of a trauma patient who needs resuscitation.
E. all of the above

_____ 49. Care for the patient with crush syndrome includes:
A. rapid transport.
B. fluid resuscitation.
C. diuresis.
D. possibly systemic alkalinization.
E. all of the above

_____ 50. The most ideal fluid for the resuscitation of the crush syndrome patient, prior to extrication, is:
A. hetastarch.
B. normal saline.
C. lactated Ringer's solution.
D. 5 percent dextrose in 1/2 normal saline.
E. Dextran.

_____ 51. It is recommended that you infuse what volume of fluid to the crush syndrome patient per hour of entrapment?
A. 200 mL
B. 400 mL
C. 500 mL
D. 600 mL
E. 1,000 mL

_____ 52. Sudden cardiac arrest care after extrication of the entrapped patient with crush syndrome should include the routine cardiac drugs and:
A. potassium for hypokalemia.
B. calcium chloride for hypokalemia.
C. sodium bicarbonate for hypokalemia.
D. dopamine for low blood pressure.
E. none of the above

_____ 53. The most prominent symptom of compartment syndrome is:
A. pain out of proportion to physical findings with the injury.
B. reduced or absent distal pulses.
C. increased skin tension in the affected limb.
D. paresthesia.
E. paresis.

_____ 54. Compartment syndrome is most likely to occur:
  A. immediately after injury.
  B. within 2 hours of injury.
  C. within 3 hours of injury.
  D. within 4 hours of injury.
  E. 6 to 8 hours after injury.

_____ 55. The most effective treatment in the prehospital setting for compartment syndrome is:
  A. a fasciectomy.
  B. the application of cold packs.
  C. elevation of the extremity.
  D. massaging the extremity.
  E. none of the above

SPECIAL PROJECT

Arterial Pressure Point—Personal Benchmarking

Locating pressure points to assist in the control of external hemorrhage is an essential skill that must be performed quickly and accurately in the emergency setting. To prepare for the possible application of this skill, locate the following pulse points on yourself. They are shown on page 98 of the textbook.

Facial artery

Brachial artery

Radial artery

Femoral artery

Popliteal artery

Medial maleolar (tibial) artery

Also practice locating these arteries on other care providers or friends. Compress the artery with one hand while monitoring the distal pulse with the other. You should notice the distal pulse strength lessening or disappearing altogether. With more distal extremities, you may notice the distal skin becoming cool and somewhat ashen.

CHAPTER 6

Burns

Review of Chapter Objectives

After reading this chapter, you should be able to:

1. **Describe the anatomy and physiology of the skin and remaining human anatomy as they pertain to thermal burn injuries.** pp. 173–175

   The skin or integumentary system is the largest organ of the body and consists of three layers, the epidermis, the dermis, and the subcutaneous layer. It functions as the outer barrier of the body and protects it against environmental extremes and pathogens. The outer-most layer is the epidermis, a layer of dead or dying cells that provides a barrier to fluid loss, absorption, and the entrance of pathogens. The dermis is the true skin. It houses the sensory nerve endings, many of the specialized skin cells that produce sweat, oil, etc., and the upper-level capillary beds that allow for the conduction of heat to the body's surface. The subcutaneous layer, although not a true part of the skin, works in concert with the skin to insulate the body from heat loss and the effects of trauma.

2. **Describe the epidemiology, including incidence, mortality/morbidity, and risk factors for thermal burn injuries as well as strategies to prevent such injuries.** pp. 172–173

   The incidence of burn injury has been declining over the past few decades but still accounts for over 1 million burn injuries and over 50,000 hospitalizations each year. Those at greatest risk are the very young, the elderly, the infirm, and those exposed to occupational risk (firefighters, chemical workers, etc.). Burns are the second leading cause of death for children under 12 and the fourth leading cause of trauma death.

   Much of the decline in burn injury and death is attributable to better building codes, improved construction techniques, and the use of smoke detectors. Educational programs that teach children not to play with matches or lighters and that instruct the family to turn the water heater down to below 130°F have also helped reduce burn morbidity and mortality.

3. **Describe the local and systemic complications of a thermal burn injury.** pp. 175–177, 187–190

   Thermal burn injury results as the rate of molecular movement in a cell increases, causing the cell membranes and proteins to denature. This causes a progressive injury as the heat penetrates deeper and deeper through the skin and into the body's interior. At the local level, the injury disrupts the envelope of the body, permitting fluid to leak from the capillaries into the tissue and evaporate, resulting in dehydration and cooling. Serious circumferential burns may form an eschar and constrict, restricting ventilation or circulation to a distal extremity.

   The systemic effects of serious burns include severe dehydration and infection. Fluid is drawn to the injured tissue as it becomes edematous and then may evaporate in great quantities as the skin loses its ability to contain fluids. Infection can be massive and can quickly and easily overwhelm the body's immune system. The products of cell destruction from the burn process may enter the bloodstream and damage the tubules of the kidneys, resulting in failure. Organ failure due to burn byproducts may also affect the liver and the heart's electrical system. Lastly, the burn injury and the associated evaporation of fluid may cool the body more rapidly than it can create heat. The result is a lowering of body temperature, hypothermia.

4. **Identify and describe the depth classifications of burn injuries, including superficial burns, partial-thickness burns, and full-thickness burns.** pp. 185–187

Superficial (first-degree) burns involve only the upper layers of the epidermis and dermis. The effects are limited to an irritation of the upper sensory tissues with some pain, minor edema, and erythema.

Partial-thickness (second-degree) burns penetrate slightly deeper than first-degree burns and cause blistering, erythema, swelling, and pain. Since the cells that reproduce the skin's upper layers are still alive, complete regeneration is expected.

Full-thickness (third-degree) burns penetrate the entire dermis, causing extensive destruction. The burned area may display a variety of appearances and colors, the site is anesthetic, and healing is prolonged. Third-degree burns may involve not only the skin, but also underlying tissues and organs. (Organ and other tissue involvement is sometimes called fourth-degree burn)

5. **Describe and apply the "rule of nines," and the "rule of palms" methods for determining body surface area percentage of a burn injury.** pp. 186–187

The "rule of nines" approximates the body surface area burned by assigning each body region nine percent of the total. These regions include: each upper extremity, the anterior of each lower extremity, the posterior of each lower extremity, the anterior of the abdomen, the anterior thorax, the upper back, the lower back, and the entire head and neck. The remaining one percent is assigned to the genitalia. For children, the head is given 18 percent, and the lower extremities are assigned 13 1/2 percent.

The "rule of palms" method of approximating burn surface area assumes the victim's palm surface is equivalent to one percent of the total body surface area. The care provider then estimates the burn surface area by determining the number of palmar surfaces it would take to cover the wound.

6. **Identify and describe the severity of a burn including a minor burn, a moderate burn, and a critical burn.** pp. 193–195

Minor burns are those that are superficial and cover less than 50 percent of the body surface area (BSA), partial-thickness burns covering less than 15 percent of the BSA, or full-thickness burns involving less than two percent of the body surface area.

Moderate burns are classified as superficial burns over more than 50 percent of the BSA, partial-thickness burns covering less then 30 percent of the BSA; or full-thickness burns covering less than 10 percent of the BSA.

Critical burns are those partial-thickness burns covering more than 30 percent of the BSA, full-thickness burns over 10 percent of the BSA, and any significant inhalation injury. Critical burns also include any burns that involve any partial or full-thickness burn to the hands, feet, genitalia, joints, or face.

7. **Describe the effects age and pre-existing conditions have on burn severity and a patient's prognosis.** pp. 189, 194

Burn patients who are very young, very old, or have a significant pre-existing disease are at increased risk for the systemic problems associated with burn injury. They cannot tolerate massive fluid losses often associated with burns because they have smaller fluid reserves and they cannot effectively fight the ensuing massive infection commonly associated with large burns. They should be considered one step closer to critical than consideration of their burn type and BSA would normally place them.

8. Discuss complications of burn injuries caused by trauma, blast injuries, airway compromise, respiratory compromise, and child abuse.

pp. 183–185, 189–191, 198–199

Traumatic injury, in the presence of burn injury, is a complicating factor that interferes with the burn healing process and may exacerbate hypovolemia. Any time these injuries coexist, the patient should be considered a higher priority than either injury would suggest, and the paramedic must care for both conditions.

Blast mechanisms produce injury through thermal burns, the pressure wave, projectile impact, and structural collapse (crush) mechanisms. When burns coexist with these other injuries, the patient priority for care and transport must be elevated at least one priority level and all injuries must be cared for. Again, the patient will have to heal from multiple injuries, making the recovery process more difficult.

Airway and respiratory compromise associated with burn injury is an extremely serious complication. The airway must be secured early, possibly with rapid sequence intubation, and adequate ventilation with supplemental oxygen ensured. Swelling of the upper or lower airway may rapidly occlude it, preventing both ventilation and intubation. In extreme circumstances, cricothyrotomy may be required. Also be watchful for carbon monoxide poisoning as it can reduce the effectiveness of oxygen transport without overt signs.

Burns associated with child abuse often result from scalding water immersion, open flame burns, or cigarette-type injuries. The child presents with a history of a burn that does not make sense, such as stove burns when he or she cannot yet reach the stove, multiple circular burns (cigarettes), or burns isolated to the buttocks, which occur as the child lifts his or her legs during attempts at immersion in hot water.

9. Describe thermal burn management including considerations for airway and ventilation, circulation, pharmacological and nonpharmacological measures, transport decisions, and psychological support/communication strategies.

pp. 190–199

The management of the burn patient is a rather complicated, multifaceted process. The first consideration is to extinguish the fire to ensure the burn does not continue. If necessary, use water from a low-pressure hose and remove all jewelry, leather, nylon, or other material that may continue to smolder or hold heat and continue to burn the patient. Also consider removing any restrictive jewelry or clothing, as such an item may act as tourniquet, restricting distal blood flow as the burn region swells.

Then assess and assure that the airway remains adequate. With any history suggestive of an inhalation burn or injury, carefully assess and monitor the airway for any signs of restriction. If they are found, move to protect the airway with rapid sequence intubation early, before the progressive airway swelling prevents intubation or significantly restricts the size of the endotracheal tube you can introduce. Small and painful burns may be covered with wet dressings to occlude airflow and reduce the pain; however, any extensive burn should be covered with a sterile dry dressing to prevent body cooling and the introduction of pathogens through the dressing.

Resuscitation for extensive burns must include large volumes of prehospital fluid (0.5 mL/kg × BSA) as burns often account for massive fluid loss into and through the burn. The patient must also be kept warm because by their nature burns account for rapid heat loss.

Any burns on opposing tissue, such as between the fingers and toes, should be separated by nonadherent dressings, as the burned surfaces are likely to adhere firmly together and cause further damage as they are pulled apart. In painful burns consider morphine, in 2 mg increments, for pain relief as long as there is no evidence of hypotension or respiratory depression.

Watch for any constriction from eschar formation that may reduce or halt distal circulation or restrict respiration. Medical direction may request a surgical incision to relieve the pressure (an escharotomy).

Any burn patient with serious injury should be transported to the burn center where he or she can receive the specialized treatment needed. Also assure that the burn patient receives therapeutic communication while you are at the scene and during transport. The burn injury is very painful and the appearance can be very frightening. Constantly talk with the patient. Try to distract him or her from the injury, and monitor level of consciousness and anxiety level throughout your care and transport.

10. Describe special considerations for a pediatric patient with a burn injury and describe the criteria for determining pediatric burn severity.
pp. 193–195

To determine the severity of a burn for a pediatric patient, you must first examine the depth of burn (superficial, partial, or full thickness) and then determine the BSA affected. With children the head is given a greater percentage of BSA (18%) and the legs are given less (13½%). (Please note that there are several more specific methods to determine BSA for children that better take into account their changing anatomy, but they are more complicated and age- and size-specific and harder to use.) Once the BSA and depth of burn are determined, the pediatric patient is assigned a level of severity one place higher than that for the adult. Any serious burn to the airway, face, joint, hand, foot, or any circumferential burn is considered serious or critical as is the pediatric burn patient with another pre-existing disease or traumatic injury.

11. Describe the specific epidemiologies, mechanisms of injury, pathophysiologies, and severity assessments for inhalation, chemical, and electrical burn injuries and for radiation exposure.
pp. 177–185, 199–206

Inhalation injuries are commonly associated with burn injuries and endanger the airway. They are caused by the inhalation of hot air or flame, which cause limited damage, by superheated steam, which results in much more significant thermal damage, or by the inhalation of toxic products of combustion, which results in chemical burns. Inhalation injury can also involve carbon monoxide poisoning and the absorption of chemicals through the alveoli and systemic poisoning. Any sign of respiratory involvement during the burn assessment process is reason to consider early and aggressive airway care and rapid transport.

Chemical burn injury is most frequently found in the industrial setting and is frequently associated with the effects of strong acids or alkalis. Both mechanisms destroy cell membranes as they penetrate deeper and deeper. The nature of the wounding process is somewhat self-limiting, though alkali burns tend to penetrate more deeply. Any chemical burn that disrupts the skin should be considered serious.

Electrical burn injuries are infrequent but can be very serious. As electricity passes through body tissue, resistance creates heat energy and damage to the cell membranes. The blood vessels and nerve pathways are especially sensitive to electrical injury. The heat produced can be extremely high and cause severe and deeply internal burn injury, depending upon the voltage and current levels involved. Any electrical burn that causes external injury or any passage of significant electrical current through the body is reason to consider the patient a high priority for transport, even if no overt signs of injury exist. Electrical injury can also affect the muscles of respiration and induce hypoxia or anoxia if the current remains. Electrical disturbances can also affect the heart, producing dysrhythmias. A special electrical injury is the lightning strike. Extremely high voltage can cause extensive internal injury, though often the current passes over the exterior of the body, resulting in limited damage. Resuscitation of the patient struck by lightning should be prolonged as this mechanism of injury may permit survival after lengthy resuscitation.

Radiation exposure is a relatively rare injury process caused by the passage of radiation energy through body cells. The radiation changes the structure of molecules and may cause cells to die, dysfunction, or reproduce dysfunctional cells. Radiation hazards cannot be seen, heard, or felt, yet they can cause both immediate and long-term health problems and death. The objective of rescue and care is to limit the exposure for both the patient and rescuer. Radiation exposure is cumulative. The less time in an area of hazard, the less effect radiation will have on the human body. The greater the distance from a radiation source, the less strength and potential it has to cause damage. Radiation levels are diminished as the particles travel through dense objects. By placing more mass between the source and patient and rescuers, the exposure is reduced. Since it is very difficult to determine the extent of exposure, gather what information you can and transport the patient for further evaluation.

12. Discuss special considerations that impact the assessment, management, and prognosis of patients with inhalation, chemical, and electrical burn injuries and with exposure to radiation.   pp. 199–206

When assessing an inhalation injury, you should examine the mechanism of injury to identify any unconsciousness or confinement during fire or any history of explosive stream expansion and inhalation. Study the patient carefully for signs of facial burns, carbonaceous sputum, or any hoarseness. Should there be any reason to suspect inhalation injury, monitor the airway very carefully and consider oxygen therapy and early intubation (RSI) as needed. The airway tissues can swell quickly and result in serious airway restriction or complete obstruction.

Chemical burn injury is indicated by the signs or history of such exposure and should begin with an identification of the agent and type of exposure. Remove contaminated clothing and dispose of it properly. The site of exposure should be irrigated with copious amounts of cool water and, once the chemical is completely removed, covered with a dry sterile dressing. Special consideration should be given to contact with phenol (soluble in alcohol), dry lime (brush off before irrigation), sodium metal (cover with oil to prevent combustion), and riot control agents (emotional support). The prognosis for a serious chemical burn is related to the agent, length of exposure to it, and depth of damage. These injuries are often severe and will leave damaged or scar tissue behind.

With an electrical burn injury, direct your assessment to seeking out and examining entrance and exit wounds and to trying to determine the voltage and current of the source. The wounds should be covered with dry sterile dressings and the patient monitored for dysrhythmias. Even if the entrance and exit wounds seem minor, consider this patient for rapid transport as the internal injury may be extensive.

Radiation is invisible and otherwise undetectable by human senses. When radiation exposure is suspected, ensure that you and the patient remain as remote from the source (distance) with as much matter as possible between you and the source (shielding) and that you spend as little time close to the source as possible. Attention to these factors will reduce the amount of radiologic exposure for both you and the patient. Assessment of the patient exposed to a radiation source is very difficult because the signs of injury are delayed except in cases of extreme exposure. Any suggestion of exposure to radiation merits examination at the emergency department and assessment of the risk by specially trained experts in the field. Limited radiation exposure does not often result in medical problems, but more severe doses may cause sterility or, later in life, cancer. Extensive exposure may cause severe illness or death.

13. Differentiate between supraglottic and infraglottic inhalation burn injuries.   pp. 183–185

A supraglottic inhalation burn is a thermal injury to the mucosa above the glottic opening. It is a significant burn because the tissue is very vascular and will swell very quickly and extensively. Because of the moist environment and the vascular nature of the tissue, it takes great heat energy to cause burn injury. When such injury occurs, however, the associated swelling can quickly threaten the airway.

Infraglottic (or subglottic) inhalation burns occur much less frequently because the moist supraglottic tissue absorbs the heat energy and the glottis will likely close to prevent the injury from penetrating more deeply. However, superheated steam, as is produced when a stream of water hits a particularly hot portion of a fire, has the heat energy to carry the burning process to the subglottic region. There, airway burns are extremely critical, as even slight tissue swelling will restrict the airway.

Special consideration should also be given to the toxic nature of the hot gasses inhaled during the inhalation burn. Modern construction materials and the widespread use of synthetics are products that release toxic agents when they burn (cyanide, arsenic, hydrogen sulfide, and others). Often these agents will combine with the moisture of the airway and form caustic compounds that induce chemical burns of the airway, or they may be absorbed into the bloodstream, causing systemic poisoning. The risk for inhalation injury increases with a history of unconsciousness or with being within a confined space during a fire.

14. Describe the special considerations for a chemical burn injury to the eye.   pp. 201–203

Chemicals introduced onto the surface of the eye threaten to damage the delicate corneal surface. It is imperative that you consider these injuries when chemicals are splashed and that the eye is irrigated for up to 20 minutes. Irrigation may be accomplished by running normal saline through an administration set into the corner of the eye and directed away from the other eye if it is not affected. If both eyes are involved, a nasal cannula may be helpful in directing fluid flow to both eyes simultaneously. Be alert for contact lenses, as they may trap chemicals under their surface and prevent effective irrigation.

15. Given several scenarios involving thermal, inhalation, electrical, and chemical burn injury and radiation exposure patients, provide the appropriate assessment and field management.   pp. 190–206

During your training as an EMT-Paramedic you will participate in many classroom practice sessions involving simulated patients. You will also spend some time in the emergency departments of local hospitals as well as in advanced-level ambulances gaining clinical experience. During these times, use your knowledge of burn trauma to help you assess and care for the simulated or real patients you attend.

CASE STUDY REVIEW

Reread the case study on pages 171 and 172 in Paramedic Care: Trauma Emergencies *before reading the discussion below.*

The scenario presented in this case study illustrates the dangers associated with the fire-ground and with inhalation injuries. It also identifies the difficulty you might have in recognizing respiratory injury and the importance of treating it early.

The scene observed by Ben and Ronny demonstrates the dangers associated with a working fire and a real-time assessment of the mechanism of injury. As Fire Rescue paramedics, they are wearing turnout gear, boots, and heavy gloves as they approach the injured firefighter. They ensure that the scene is safe and recognize that hazards can include debris, still energized electrical lines, leaking gas, further structural collapse, and much more. They will work quickly to move their fellow firefighter to a safe location and continue care. Once at a safe location, Ben and Ronny remove the firefighter's clothing as they begin their initial assessment. They replace their work gloves with sterile latex or plastic ones because they well know that infection is a common and serious consequence of the types of burns this patient received. They will do all they can to protect the wounds from further contamination by quickly covering them with dry sterile dressings.

The firefighter they assess in this incident experiences the classic evolution of the burn and inhalation injury. He was initially found to be stable with signs, symptoms, and vital signs suggestive of minor injury. The major concern for this patient might well be the fractured forearm. However, the paramedics are wary because of the significant area burned and the patient's history, hoarseness, and the sooty sputum. They anticipate serious fluid loss through the burn and infection risk as well as airway injury that will likely worsen during their care.

Ben must be careful regarding any articles of clothing or jewelry that could continue to burn or contain the swelling that often accompanies burn injury. His initial action should be to stop any further burning. This calls for complete inspection of the burn area and the surrounding clothing. Once the burn area is exposed, the depth and area involved can be assessed. In this case, the patient has a fracture, possible inhalation injury, and a serious burn. The area burned, the posterior chest and abdomen and the upper left extremity, represent a body surface area of about 22 1/2 percent. The combination of traumatic injury, burn, and inhalation injury are reasons to consider the patient to have critical injuries.

The paramedics initiate an IV with a large-bore catheter and begin running normal saline. A 1,000 mL bag is hung with a non-flow-restrictive (trauma or blood tubing) administration set just in case the signs of shock appear. Fluids are run rapidly to get ahead of the loss normally associated with severe burns. If this were a 125 kg man with the burns identified (22 1/2% by the rule of nines), the needed fluid would be 4 mL × 22½ (percent of burn area) × 125 kg or a total of 11,250 mL in the first 24 hours (Parkland formula). Half of this is needed in the first 8 hours. That's more than 700 mL per hour.

The signs of respiratory involvement, though subtle, are even more significant than the burn or fracture. Inhalation injury is likely due either to the chemical burning caused by the products of combustion reacting with the soft tissue of the respiratory tract or to thermal burns caused by superheated steam created when the water extinguished the flames. In either case, respiratory damage can be extensive. Patients with respiratory burns usually display progressive dyspnea, as in this case. The only effective way to treat this problem is to anticipate that progression and be aggressive in airway care. Intubation equipment should be readied and used when any sign of developing airway compromise appears. With inhalation injury it might be prudent to consider rapid sequence intubation to allow the passage of the endotracheal tube before the airway swells and makes the procedure very difficult. Ken should also be considered for immediate transport because of the difficulty in managing the airway.

Ben and Ronny must also be prepared for the worst. If the firefighter had experienced severe dyspnea and airway restriction while 20 to 30 minutes from the hospital, a needle or surgical cricothyrotomy might have been necessary. Likewise, had they waited on the scene to splint, bandage, and care for the patient, the time spent on those tasks would have permitted the airway and patient to deteriorate. This case study clearly identifies the need for rapid recognition and transport of the patient with developing airway compromise.

CONTENT SELF-EVALUATION

MULTIPLE CHOICE

_____ 1. The incidence of burn injury has been on the decline over the past decade.
 A. True
 B. False

_____ 2. A preventative action that will reduce the incidence of scalding injuries is:
 A. use of child-proof faucets.
 B. education of children on the dangers of hot water.
 C. placing caution stickers on water faucets.
 D. lowering the water heater temperature to 130°F.
 E. none of the above

_____ 3. The layer of skin that is made up of mostly dead cells and provides the waterproof envelope that contains the body is the:
 A. dermis.   D. sebum.
 B. subcutaneous layer.   E. corium.
 C. epidermis.

_____ 4. Which of the following is NOT a function of the skin?
 A. protecting the body from bacterial infection
 B. protecting the body from excessive fluid loss
 C. allowing for joint movement
 D. prevention of all heat loss
 E. insulating from trauma

_____ 5. Burns result from the disruption of the proteins found in cell membranes.
 A. True
 B. False

_____ 6. The area of a burn that suffers the most damage is generally the:
 A. the zone of hyperemia.   D. the zone of coagulation.
 B. the zone of denaturing.   E. the zone of most resistance.
 C. the zone of stasis.

_____ 7. The theory of burns that explains the burning process is:
A. the thermal hypothesis.
B. Jackson's theory of thermal wounds.
C. the Phaseal discussion of burns.
D. the Hypermetabolism dynamic.
E. none of the above

_____ 8. The order in which the phases of the body's response to a burn would normally be expected to occur is:
A. emergent, fluid shift, hypermetabolic
B. fluid shift, hypermetabolic, emergent
C. fluid shift, emergent, hypermetabolic
D. hypermetabolic, fluid shift, emergent
E. emergent, hypermetabolic, fluid shift

_____ 9. Which of the following skin types has the greatest resistance to the passage of electrical current?
A. mucous membranes
B. wet skin
C. calluses
D. the skin on the inside of the arm
E. the skin on the inside of the thigh

_____ 10. Electrical injury is likely to cause which of the following?
A. serious injury where the electricity enters the body
B. serious injury where the electricity exits the body
C. damage to nerves
D. damage to blood vessels
E. all of the above

_____ 11. Prolonged contact with alternating current may result in respiratory paralysis.
A. True
B. False

_____ 12. Chemical burns involving strong alkalis are likely to be deep due to coagulation necrosis.
A. True
B. False

_____ 13. Which of the following radiation types is the most powerful type of ionizing radiation?
A. lambda
B. alpha
C. gamma
D. beta
E. delta

_____ 14. Which of the following is a type of radiation present only inside nuclear reactors and bombs?
A. neutron
B. alpha
C. gamma
D. beta
E. delta

_____ 15. To protect themselves from radiation exposure, EMS personnel should:
A. limit the duration of exposure.
B. increase the shielding from exposure.
C. increase the distance from the source.
D. ensure that the patient is decontaminated.
E. all of the above

_____ 16. The radiation dose that is lethal to about 50 percent of those exposed is:
A. 0.2 Gray.
B. 100 rads.
C. 1 Gray.
D. 4.5 Grays.
E. 200 rads.

_____ 17. As radiation exposure increases, the signs of exposure become less evident and only reappear later in the course of the disease.
A. True
B. False

_____ 18. Which of the following is commonly associated with inhalation injury?
A. carbon monoxide poisoning
B. toxic inhalation
C. supraglottic injury
D. subglottic injury
E. all of the above

_____ 19. Which type of circumstance is most likely to cause subglottic thermal burn injury?
A. inhalation of hot air
B. inhalation of flame
C. inhalation of superheated steam
D. standing in a burn environment
E. inhalation of toxic substances

_____ 20. What percentage of burn patients who die have associated airway burn injury?
A. 20 percent
B. 35 percent
C. 50 percent
D. 60 percent
E. 80 percent

_____ 21. The burn characterized by erythema, pain, and blistering is the:
A. superficial burn.
B. partial-thickness burn.
C. full-thickness burn.
D. electrical burn.
E. chemical burn.

_____ 22. The burn characterized by discoloration and lack of pain is the:
A. superficial burn.
B. partial-thickness burn.
C. full-thickness burn.
D. electrical burn.
E. chemical burn.

_____ 23. An adult has received burns to the entire anterior chest and to the entire left upper extremity, circumferentially. Using the rule of nines, the percentage of body surface (BSA) area involved is:
A. 9 percent.
B. 18 percent.
C. 27 percent.
D. 36 percent.
E. 48 percent.

_____ 24. A child has received burns to the entire left lower extremity and the genitals. Using the rule of nines, the percentage of the body surface area involved is:
A. 9 percent.
B. 10 percent.
C. $14^{1/2}$ percent.
D. 19 percent.
E. $21^{1/2}$ percent.

_____ 25. An adult has received burns to the entire left lower extremity and the genitals. Using the rule of nines, the percentage of the body surface area involved is:
A. 9 percent.
B. 10 percent.
C. 18 percent.
D. 19 percent.
E. 21 percent.

_____ 26. A child receives burns to his entire head and neck and upper back. What percentage of body surface area is involved?
A. 9 percent
B. 10 percent
C. 18 percent
D. 19 percent
E. 27 percent

_____ 27. Which of the following systemic complications should you suspect with all serious burns?
A. hypothermia
B. hypovolemia
C. infection
D. eschar formation
E. all of the above

_____ 28. Which of the following conditions would increase the impact a burn has on a patient?
- **A.** being very young
- **B.** being very old
- **C.** having the flu
- **D.** emphysema
- **E.** all of the above

_____ 29. Which of the following should NOT be removed from any burned area of a patient?
- **A.** nylon clothing such as a windbreaker
- **B.** small pieces of burned fabric lodged in the wound
- **C.** shoes and socks
- **D.** rings, watches, and other articles of jewelry
- **E.** leather belts

_____ 30. When considering intubation of the patient with suspected airway injury due to inhalation of the byproducts of combustion, you should have a several smaller than normal endotracheal tubes ready.
- **A.** True
- **B.** False

_____ 31. In severe inhalation injury due to airway burns it may be necessary to perform a cricothyrotomy to secure an adequate airway.
- **A.** True
- **B.** False

_____ 32. High-flow oxygen therapy is very helpful in cases of carbon monoxide poisoning because it will then be carried in sufficient quantities in the plasma to maintain life.
- **A.** True
- **B.** False

_____ 33. Your assessment reveals an area of burn that is reddened, painful, and just beginning to display blisters. What burn classification would you give this burn?
- **A.** superficial burn
- **B.** partial-thickness burn
- **C.** full-thickness burn
- **D.** first degree burn
- **E.** A or D

_____ 34. The patient you are attending has her entire left upper extremity seriously burned. The forearm and hand are very painful and reddened, while the upper arm is relatively painless and a dark red color. What percentage of the BSA and burn depth would you assign this patient?
- **A.** 9 percent full-thickness burn
- **B.** 9 percent partial-thickness burn
- **C.** 4 1/2 percent full-thickness burn
- **D.** 4 1/2 percent partial-thickness burn
- **E.** 4 1/2 percent partial-thickness and 4 1/2 percent full-thickness burn

_____ 35. Your assessment reveals a burn patient with superficial burns to 27 percent of the body. To which classification of burn severity would you assign her?
- **A.** minor
- **B.** moderate
- **C.** serious
- **D.** critical
- **E.** none of the above

_____ 36. Your assessment reveals a burn patient with full-thickness burns to the entire left thigh and calf. What classification of burn severity would you assign him?
- **A.** minor
- **B.** moderate
- **C.** serious
- **D.** critical
- **E.** none of the above

_____ 37. Your assessment reveals a burn patient with partial-thickness burns to all of both lower extremities. What classification of burn severity would you assign her?
- **A.** minor
- **B.** moderate
- **C.** serious
- **D.** critical
- **E.** none of the above

_____ 38. Your assessment reveals a burn patient with partial-thickness burns to her entire lower extremities and a suspected femur fracture. What classification of burn severity would you assign her?
A. minor
B. moderate
C. serious
D. critical
E. none of the above

_____ 39. Cool water immersion may reduce the depth and significance of small burns if applied within:
A. 1 to 2 minutes.
B. 2 to 4 minutes.
C. 4 to 5 minutes.
D. 10 minutes.
E. 20 minutes.

_____ 40. The patient with any full-thickness burn should be considered for administration of tetanus toxoid as the wound is an open one.
A. True
B. False

_____ 41. In general, moderate to severe burns should be covered with:
A. moist occlusive dressings.
B. dry sterile dressings.
C. cool water immersion.
D. plastic wrap covered by a soft dressing.
E. warm water immersion.

_____ 42. Adjacent full-thickness burns, such as those affecting the fingers and toes, should be held together without dressings to ensure rapid healing.
A. True
B. False

_____ 43. The Parkland formula for fluid administration calls for administration of 4 mL of fluid to a patient multiplied by the patient's BSA involved. What other factor(s) determines the total fluid administered in the first 24 hours?
A. patient's age
B. patient's weight
C. depth of burns
D. age of the patient
E. all of the above

_____ 44. Which of the following is the preferred fluid for resuscitation of the severely burned patient?
A. normal saline
B. 1/2 normal saline
C. dextrose 5 percent in water
D. lactated Ringer's solution
E. dextrose 5 percent in normal saline

_____ 45. Which of the following drugs may be given to the patient with severe burns in the prehospital setting?
A. ipratropium
B. morphine
C. epinephrine
D. furosemide
E. haloperidol

_____ 46. Which of the following may be appropriate when a forming eschar is restricting distal blood flow to an extremity?
A. elevating the extremity
B. incising the eschar to relieve the pressure
C. wrapping the extremity in dry sterile dressings
D. administering morphine
E. immersing the limb in cold water

_____ 47. A patient was found unconscious in a burning mobile home. Your assessment discovers severe dyspnea, no airway restriction, chest pain, altered mental status, and some seizure activity. What condition would you suspect?
A. carbon monoxide poisoning
B. cyanide poisoning
C. chemical burns to the lungs
D. hypoxia due to inhalation of oxygen-deprived air
E. superheated steam inhalation

_____ 48. If an IV line is not yet established in a patient with suspected cyanide poisoning you should administer which of the following?
   A. amyl nitrate
   B. sodium nitrate
   C. sodium thiosulfide
   D. haloperidol
   E. ipratropium

_____ 49. In addition to the entrance and exit wounds normally expected with the passage of electrical current through the human body, the paramedic should expect:
   A. ventricular fibrillation.
   B. cardiac irritability.
   C. internal damage.
   D. smoldering clothing.
   E. all of the above

_____ 50. In the United States, lightning strikes hit about how many people per year?
   A. 25
   B. 50
   C. 100
   D. 300
   E. 500

_____ 51. The patient who is unresponsive, apneic, and pulseless due to a lightning strike is not a likely candidate for successful resuscitation.
   A. True
   B. False

_____ 52. In general, caustic chemical contamination should be cared for by:
   A. dry sterile dressings.
   B. chemical antidotes.
   C. rigorous scrubbing.
   D. cool water irrigation.
   E. rapid transport.

_____ 53. The chemical phenol is soluble in:
   A. water.
   B. dry lime.
   C. normal saline.
   D. ammonia.
   E. none of the above

_____ 54. Which chemical agent reacts vigorously with water?
   A. phenol
   B. bleach
   C. sodium
   D. riot control agents
   E. ammonia

_____ 55. Known antidotes and neutralizers for chemical contamination and burns will reduce the injury caused by the agent if administered immediately.
   A. True
   B. False

_____ 56. How long should you irrigate a patient's eye contaminated with chemicals of an unknown nature?
   A. less than 2 minutes
   B. up to 5 minutes
   C. up to 15 minutes
   D. up to 20 minutes
   E. none of the above

_____ 57. When chemicals are splashed into the eye of the patient wearing contact lenses, the contact should be removed to ensure irrigation will remove all of the agent.
   A. True
   B. False

_____ 58. If the source of radiation cannot be contained or moved away from the patient:
   A. the patient should be brought to you.
   B. care should be offered by you in protective gear.
   C. care should be offered by specialists in protective gear.
   D. care should be offered by the highest ranking officer.
   E. A or C

_____ 59. Which action can be used reduce rescuer exposure to a radiation source?
   A. increase the distance from the source
   B. decrease the time exposed to the source
   C. increase the shielding between the rescuer and source
   D. protect against inhalation of contaminated dust
   E. all of the above

_____ 60. Once exposed to a significant radiation source, the patient will become a source of radiation that the rescuer must then protect him- or herself against. No amount of decontamination will reduce this danger.
   A. True
   B. False

SPECIAL PROJECT

Drip Math Worksheet 2

Formulas
Rate = Volume/Time   mL/min = gtts per min/gtts per mL
Volume = Rate × Time   gtts/min = mL per min × gtts per mL
Time = Volume/Rate   mL = gtts/gtts per mL

Please complete the following drip math problems:

1. You are asked to administer a 250 mL solution to a patient over 2 hours. What drip rate would you use with a:

   A. 10 gtts per mL administration set

   B. 15 gtts per mL administration set

   C. 60 gtts per mL administration set

2. Your protocol directs that an IV drip is to be run at 30 gtts per minute with a 60 gtts per mL administration set. How long will it take to infuse:

A. 200 ml

B. 350 ml

3. How much fluid would you administer to a patient over 15 minutes with a macrodrip (15 gtts/mL) administration set, running at 1 gtt per second?

4. Your protocol requires you to administer a drug at 15 gtts per minute with a 60 gtts per mL administration set. You only have a 45 gtts per mL set available. What drip rate would you run it at?

CHAPTER 7

Musculoskeletal Trauma

Review of Chapter Objectives

After reading this chapter, you should be able to:

1. Describe the incidence, morbidity, and mortality of musculoskeletal injuries.   pp. 210–211

In trauma, musculoskeletal injuries are second in frequency only to soft-tissue injuries. They account for millions of injuries ranging from strains to fractures and dislocations and are rarely, by themselves, life threatening. However, significant musculoskeletal injuries are found in 80 percent of patients who suffer multi-system trauma and may account for significant disability.

2. Discuss the anatomy and physiology of the muscular and skeletal systems.   pp. 211–224

The skeletal system is a living body system that protects vital organs, acts as a storehouse for body salts and other materials needed for metabolism, produces erythrocytes, permits us to have an upright stature, and permits us to move with relative ease through the environment. The skeletal system consists of the axial and appendicular skeletons.

The common long bone consists of a diaphysis, metaphysis, and epiphysis. The diaphysis is the hollow skeletal shaft of the long bone and contains the yellow bone marrow. It is covered by the periosteum, which contains sensory nerve fibers and initiates the bone repair cycle. The metaphysis is the transitional region between the diaphysis and the epiphysis. In this region, the thin layer of compact bone of the diaphysis shaft becomes the honeycomb of the weight-bearing epiphyseal region. The epiphysis is the articular end of the bone. Through the widening of the metaphysis and the cancellous bone underneath, the weight-bearing, articular surface distributes support over a large surface area.

Bones join at an area called a joint, where they move together to permit articulation. The actual surface of movement is the articular surface and is covered with cartilage, a smooth, shock-absorbing surface that allows free movement between the two ends of the adjoining bones. It is the actual joint surface. The joint is held together with ligaments, which are bands of connective tissue attaching bones to each other. These bands encapsulate the joint and allow some stretch, while holding the articulating bones firmly together.

Muscles make up most of the body's mass, are the driving power behind body motion, and also provide most of the body's heat energy. They only have the ability to contract with force, hence are usually paired with one opposing the motion of the other. Muscles are usually attached by strong connective tissue called tendons. The point of attachment that remains stationary with muscle contraction is the origin, while the point of attachment that moves is the insertion.

3. Predict injuries based on the mechanism of injury, including: pp. 224–230

- **Direct.** Direct injury can be caused by blunt or penetrating mechanisms that deliver kinetic energy to the location of injury and may account for fractures, dislocations, muscle contusions, strains, sprains, subluxations, or combinations of the above.
- **Indirect.** Indirect injuries are injuries that occur as energy is transmitted along the musculoskeletal system to a point of weakness. For example: A person falls forward and braces the fall

on an outstretched arm. The energy is transmitted up the extremity to the clavicle, where a fracture occurs. Another example is the football player whose cleated shoe remains stationary while contact with an opposing player turns his body, resulting in an injury to the ligament of the knee.

- **Pathologic.** Pathologic injury results from tumors of the periosteum, bone, articular cartilage, ligaments, tendons, or muscles. Diseases that affect the musculoskeletal structures may also cause injuries as may radiation treatment. Bones or joint structures injured in this way are not likely to heal well.

4. **Discuss the types of musculoskeletal injuries, including:**

- **Fractures (open and closed)**   **pp. 227–229**
  A fracture is a break in the continuity of the bone. It may present with pain, false motion, angulation, and, possibly, an open wound.

- **Dislocations/fractures**   **pp. 226–227**
  A dislocation is a displacement of one of the bones of a joint from the joint capsule. The area is noticeably deformed, the limb is usually fixed in position, and the injury is very painful. Due to the proximity of blood vessels and nerves, there is a concern for involvement of these structures and loss of distal circulation and sensation. A fracture is a disruption in the continuity of a bone. In a closed fracture, bone ends do not penetrate the skin. In an open fracture, they do. Other types of fractures include hairline, impacted, transverse, oblique, comminuted, spiral, fatigue, greenstick, and epiphyseal. Fractures may also occur in the proximity of joints and present in a similar fashion with similar dangers.

- **Sprains**   **p. 226**
  A sprain is the tearing of the ligaments of a joint. The injury produces pain, swelling, and discoloration with time. Since the injury has damaged the joint's integrity, further exertion may cause joint failure. A subluxation is a transitional injury between the sprain and dislocation. The ligaments have been stretched and do not provide a stable joint. The range of motion may be limited and the site is very painful.

- **Strains**   **p. 226**
  A strain is an overstretching of a muscle body that produces pain. The muscle fibers have been damaged; however, there is usually no internal hemorrhage or associated discoloration.

5. **Describe the six "Ps" of musculoskeletal injury assessment.**   **p. 235**

Pain. The patient with musculoskeletal injury may report pain, pain on touch (tenderness), or pain on movement of the injured limb.
Pallor. The skin at the injury site and distal to it may be pale or flushed and capillary refill may be delayed.
Paralysis. The patient may be unable to move the limb and/or may have diminished strength distal to the injury.
Paresthesia. The patient may complain of numbness or tingling or may have limited or no sensation distal to the injury.
Pressure. The patient may complain of a sensation of pressure at the site of injury or palpation may detect a greater skin tone and tissue rigidity at the injury site.
Pulses. The distal pulses may be diminished or absent distal to the injury site.

6. **List the primary signs and symptoms of extremity trauma.**   **pp. 232–237**

The primary signs of extremity trauma include pain, mechanism of injury, deformity (angulation or swelling), soft-tissue injuries (suggesting injury beneath), unusual limb placement, inequality in limb length, and the inability of the patient to bear weight or use the extremity.

7. **List other signs and symptoms that can indicate less obvious extremity injury.**   **pp. 235–238**

In addition to the six "Ps" of musculoskeletal injury, the injury may demonstrate instability of the joint or limb, inequality of sensation or limb strength, crepitus (a grating sensation), unusual motion, abnormal muscle tone, and unusual regions of warmth or coolness.

8. Discuss the need for assessment of pulses, motor function, and sensation before and after splinting. p. 241

It is essential to monitor distal pulses, sensation, and motor function during the splinting process. You need to first determine a baseline to ensure that the distal function of the limb is intact before you begin the process. If not, minor movement of the limb may restore it. Once the process is complete, and frequently thereafter, you need to ensure that the splint does not constrict the limb too forcibly, restricting distal blood flow. The check will also assure venous return is adequate and that the nerves remain uncompressed and functional.

9. Identify the circumstances requiring rapid intervention and transport when dealing with musculoskeletal injuries. pp. 233–234

Because musculoskeletal injuries are not often associated with life-threatening injuries, they by themselves do not frequently require rapid intervention and transport. However, when the distal circulation or innervation is interrupted by the injury, immediate intervention and rapid transport may be indicated. If a distal pulse or nervous function deficit is noted, you may try to gently manipulate the injury site to restore pulse or function (this includes dislocation reduction in some circumstances). It is also imperative to bring the patient to the emergency department quickly if your attempts to correct the circulation or nervous problem are unsuccessful.

10. Discuss the general guidelines for splinting. pp. 239–244

Once any patient life threats and serious injuries have been cared for, splinting may take place. The injury is assessed as are the distal pulse, sensation, and motor function. Any open wound is covered with a sterile dressing and the limb is positioned for splinting, as long as the injury is no closer than 3 inches from a joint. Provide any movement for limb positioning with gentle in-line traction unless the movement significantly increases pain or resistance is felt. Choose a device (long padded board splint, air splint, traction splint, etc.) that accommodates the limb and secure it to immobilize the joint above and the joint below the injury. Secure the splint from the distal to the proximal end to assure the best venous return and check distal circulation, sensation, and motor function in the limb at the end of the splinting process. Joint injuries are generally immobilized as found unless there is distal pulse, sensation, or motor function deficit. Then an attempt to align the injury may be indicated.

11. Explain the benefits of the application of cold and heat for musculoskeletal injuries. pp. 246, 255–257

The application of cold to a musculoskeletal injury in the few hours after the injury constricts the vasculature and limits edema. This assures better circulation through the limb after the injury, especially if splinting is employed. Heat applied after 48 hours will increase the circulation to the injury site and speed the healing process.

12. Describe age-associated changes in the bones. p. 230

As bones develop in the fetus they are almost exclusively cartilaginous in nature. This makes them extremely flexible but not very rigid. With the newborn and infants, the cartilage begins to fill with salt deposits and becomes stronger and more rigid. It is, however, still very flexible and one reason infants have a hard time standing and holding their heads up. Bones lengthen from the epiphyseal plate near the bone ends, an area where fracture may disrupt the growth process. With increasing age, children's bones become more rigid, but they are prone to fractures like the greenstick, breaking and splintering on one side but not breaking completely. By the late teen years, the bone tissue reaches its maximum strength. As an adult reaches 40 years of age, bone degeneration begins. The bones become less flexible and more prone to fracture. They also heal more slowly. With advancing age and continuing bone degeneration, fractures may occur with normal stresses and lead to falls.

13. **Discuss the pathophysiology, assessment findings, and management of open and closed fractures.** pp. 227–229, 232–250

Fractures are generally traumatic events that disrupt the structure of the bone. They may be a result of blunt trauma such as a fall or an auto collision or of penetrating trauma as when a bullet slams into a rib. Assessment will reveal a patient who complains of pain and the inability to use the extremity. Physical assessment will reveal angulation, swelling, deformity, and false motion (where joint-like motion is unexpected). Distally, the limb may display pallor, coolness, diminished or absent pulses, reduced sensation or motor function, and may be shortened when compared to the opposing limb. By definition, there will be an open wound associated with an open fracture, though it may be caused by the offending force causing the fracture or by one or more of the fractured bone ends penetrating the skin. Management includes covering any open wound with a sterile dressing and then gently aligning the bone with traction and immobilizing it and the joints above and below the injury with a splinting device.

14. **Discuss the relationship between the volume of hemorrhage and open or closed fractures.** pp. 234, 246–247

Fractures alone, whether open or closed, do not often account for severe and continued blood loss with the exception of pelvic and femoral fractures. Pelvic fractures may account for more than 2,000 mL of blood loss and femoral fractures, up to 1,500mL. Tibial/fibular and humeral fractures may account for 500mL of loss, and other fractures and dislocations for less. These losses do contribute to hypovolemia and shock in the multi-system trauma patient. Closed fractures have limited blood loss because of fascial containment of the hemorrhage, with the exception of the pelvis, where lack of any fascial compartment helps account for the severe hemorrhage associated with that injury. Open wounds may permit blood to be lost externally in excess of the numbers above, but hemorrhage control techniques should easily control that loss.

15. **Discuss the indications and contraindications for use of the pneumatic anti-shock garment (PASG) in the management of fractures.** pp. 246–247

Use of the PASG is indicated in fractures of the pelvis because of its ability to immobilize the pelvis and lower extremities and its ability to apply pressure to the abdomen and lower extremities, thereby limiting the blood loss associated with such injuries. The PASG may also be indicated in the stabilization of the patient with bilateral femur fracture for the same reasons. Contraindications include any isolated femur fracture because the traction splint provides preferred immobilization. The PASG should not be used with hip dislocations and for any fractures more distal than three inches above the knee.

16. **Describe the special considerations involved in femur fracture management.** pp. 247–248

The femur is the largest long bone of the body and its fracture requires great energy, resulting in a serious and very traumatic injury. The injury is generally very painful, causing the large muscles of the thigh to contract and naturally splint the site. This action pushes the broken femur ends into the muscles of the thigh, increasing the pain and causing further muscle spasm. The result is a serious and progressing injury. Gentle traction can prevent further damage and pain from the femur movement and then relax the muscle masses, allowing the femur ends to move back to a more anatomic position. This enhances blood flow through the limb and reduces soft tissue injury caused by the overriding bones. Gentle traction is applied manually and then is maintained by a traction splint device.

17. **Discuss the pathophysiology, assessment findings, and management of dislocations.** pp. 250–254

Dislocations are forceful events that displace the bone ends from their proper location within a joint by stretching or tearing ligaments. The patient will complain of pain and the inability to use the joint, while you will notice deformity of the joint and unusual limb placement. Dislocations are usually immobilized as they are found unless the distal pulse, sensation, or motor function distal to the injury is disrupted or the time from injury to care at the emergency department will be long. Then attempts made at dislocation reduction may be made.

18. Discuss the out-of-hospital management of dislocation/fractures, including splinting and realignment. pp. 244–254

The objective of dislocation and fracture care is splinting to prevent further injury during transport to the emergency department. A splint should be chosen for ease in application, ability to immobilize the fracture or dislocation site (and the joint above and below), and patient comfort. The limb should be aligned to ensure adequate immobilization with the splint by bringing the distal limb in line (using gentle traction) with the proximal limb. The movement continues until the limb is aligned, you meet resistance, or the patient experiences a significant increase in pain. The devices below should be utilized only if they can accomplish the goals of splinting effectively.

Pelvis—PASG, long spine board with additional support
Hip—long spine board, orthopedic stretcher
Femur—traction splint
Knee—padded board splints
Tibia and fibula—padded board splints, air splint
Ankle—pillow splint, padded board splint, air splint
Foot—pillow splint, padded board splint, air splint, conforming splint
Shoulder—sling and swathe
Humerus—cuff and collar sling and swathe
Elbow—padded board splint
Radius and ulna—padded board splint, air splint
Wrist—padded board splint, air splint
Hand—padded board splint, conforming splint, air splint
Finger—conforming splint, padded board splint

19. Explain the importance of manipulating a knee dislocation/fracture with an absent distal pulse. pp. 239–240, 244–245, 251–252

The absence of distal pulses secondary to a fracture or dislocation may be due to associated pressure on the artery due to bone displacement. Gentle, controlled manipulation may move the bones enough to re-establish the distal circulation and ensure the distal tissues receive adequate perfusion during the remaining care and transport.

20. Describe the procedure for reduction of a shoulder, finger, or ankle dislocation/fracture. pp. 252–254

The general process for dislocation reduction is to use increasing traction to move the bone ends apart (distraction) and then toward a normal anatomic position. The pull is slowly increased over about 3 minutes or until you feel the bone ends "pop" into position and see the limb assume a more normal anatomic appearance. The distal circulation, sensation, and motor function are examined before and after the procedure to ensure that distal function remains normal. Generally, reduction is not attempted unless there is serious neurovascular compromise. If the procedure does not produce relocation in a few minutes, splint the limb as is and transport.

Shoulder dislocations are most commonly anterior (hollow or squared-off shoulder) or posterior (elbow and forearm held off the chest). Place a strap across the chest and under the arm and have a rescuer pull traction against the traction you pull along the arm while you draw the arm somewhat away from the chest (abduction). Some rotation along the axis of the humerus (by rotating the elbow) may facilitate reduction. For the less common inferior dislocation, have one rescuer stabilize the chest while you flex the elbow and apply a firm traction along the axis of the humerus. Gently rotate the humerus externally.

Finger dislocations are relatively common and most often displace posteriorly. Grasp the finger and apply firm distal traction, distracting the two bone ends and moving the finger toward the normal anatomic position.

Ankle dislocations present with the ankle turned outward (lateral), the foot pointing upward (anterior), and the foot pointing downward (posterior). With the anterior dislocation, grasp the toe and heel and rotate the foot toward a normal orientation. With the anterior dislocation, move the foot posteriorly, while with posterior dislocations, move the foot anteriorly.

21. **Discuss the pathophysiology, assessment findings, and management of sprains, strains, and tendon injuries.** pp. 226, 254–255

Sprains generally result from the movement of a joint beyond its normal range of motion while the ligaments holding it together are stretched or torn. The patient will complain of a mechanism of injury and pain at the joint that usually increases with any attempt to move it or put weight on it. Management is centered around immobilizing the site and transporting the patient to rule out fracture (by x-ray).

Strains are overexertion injuries to the muscles where muscle fibers are torn. The particular muscle is sore, and pain will increase with attempts to use it. Care is centered around rest and reduced use of the muscle until the body can heal it.

Tendon injuries include tears or ruptures of the tendons, or the tendons may pull loose from their skeletal attachments. Injury is usually due to overexertion or to severe blunt or penetrating trauma. Care is usually directed at immobilizing the patient's affected limb in the position of function (neutral positioning) and transporting for assessment and possible surgical repair at the emergency department.

22. **Differentiate between musculoskeletal injuries based on the assessment findings and history.** pp. 232–238

It is very difficult to differentiate between muscle, joint, and long bone injuries in the prehospital setting. Hence, treat any suspected musculoskeletal injury found within 3 inches of a joint as a dislocation, splinting it as it is found unless there is a distal neurovascular deficit. In that case, reduction may be considered. Injuries affecting the limbs and more than 3 inches from the joint are considered fractures and are brought into alignment using gentle distal traction unless there is a great increase in pain or you meet resistance.

23. **Given several preprogrammed and moulaged musculoskeletal injury patients, provide the appropriate scene size-up, initial assessment, rapid trauma assessment or focused exam and history, and then provide the appropriate patient care and transport.** pp. 232–258

During your training as an EMT-Paramedic you will participate in many classroom practice sessions involving simulated patients. You will also spend some time in the emergency departments of local hospitals as well as in advanced-level ambulances gaining clinical experience. During these times, use your knowledge of musculoskeletal trauma to help you assess and care for the simulated or real patients you attend.

CASE STUDY REVIEW

Reread the case study on page 210 in Paramedic Care: Trauma Emergencies *before reading the discussion below.*

This case identifies some of the important aspects of skeletal injury assessment and care. It also presents an elderly patient, a member of a group that are common victims of long bone injuries due to skeletal degeneration associated with advancing age.

The description of the events surrounding the injury of this 91-year-old patient is typical of the geriatric hip injury. Weakened with age, the femur can no longer withstand the stresses of articulation and it fractures. (These types of fractures frequently occur on steps, where stresses on the bone are somewhat increased.) As the bone gives way, the patient usually feels it snap and then falls. Since the injury is not of traumatic origin, the internal soft-tissue damage is generally limited, and the patient may be relatively comfortable with the injury.

The initial assessment of Mary Herman reveals a hemodynamically stable elderly woman, but an otherwise healthy, patient with less pain than expected from a femur fracture. Since she is oriented and can speak well, Mark and Steffany feel that her airway and respirations are adequate. They quickly check her pulse rate and strength and move quickly to the focused trauma assessment. The assessment reveals an extremity that is aligned, but unstable, and only slightly painful. Further assessment reveals that the lower extremities have bilaterally equal distal pulses, color, temperature, sensation, and capillary refill times. This suggests that both innervation and circulation to the distal extremity are not compromised. Based on these findings, this patient is not a candidate for rapid transport and trauma center care. However, Mark and Steffany carefully monitor Mrs. Herman's extremity to detect any early signs of distal neurologic or vascular compromise. They also monitor her vital signs to track any early signs of shock because Mrs. Herman's age suggests she is not as able to compensate for blood loss as a younger adult might be. As a precaution, they initiate an IV line running "to keep open" but are ready to infuse a significant volume of fluid should the signs of shock appear.

Mark applies oxygen to assure efficient respirations and the oximeter to assure adequate oxygen delivery to the body cells. He also frequently auscultates the lung fields and evaluates respiration because emboli from the fracture site may travel there. The team also places an ECG on Mrs. Herman, as her age predisposes her to cardiac problems that may be exacerbated by this injury.

In the field of emergency care, this call might seem routine and anything but exciting. Care of minor "emergencies," especially those dealing with the elderly, are common. While to the paramedic there may be a desire to consider this call a "taxi ride," to the patient the injury threatens lifestyle and is an important life event. Mark and Steffany realize their responsibility to make Mary Herman as comfortable as possible, to provide the appropriate assessment and care, and to place emphasis on the patient's emotional support during care, packaging, and transport. She is treated with respect and consideration.

CONTENT SELF-EVALUATION

MULTIPLE CHOICE

_____ 1. Musculoskeletal injuries can include injury to:
   A. bones.
   B. tendons.
   C. ligaments.
   D. muscles.
   E. all of the above

_____ 2. Which of the following is NOT a function performed by the musculoskeletal system?
   A. vital organ protection
   B. a portion of the immune response
   C. storage of material necessary for metabolism
   D. hemopoietic activities
   E. efficient movement against gravity

_____ 3. The bone cell responsible for maintaining bone tissue is the:
   A. osteoblast.
   B. osteoclast.
   C. osteocyte.
   D. osteocrit.
   E. none of the above

_____ 4. The bone cell responsible for dissolving bone tissue is the:
   A. osteoblast.
   B. osteoclast.
   C. osteocyte.
   D. osteocrit.
   E. none of the above

_____ 5. The central portion of a long bone is called the:
   A. diaphysis.
   B. epiphysis.
   C. metaphysis.
   D. cancellous bone.
   E. compact bone.

_____ 6. The transitional area between the end and central portion of the long bone is called the:
   A. diaphysis.
   B. epiphysis.
   C. metaphysis.
   D. cancellous bone.
   E. compact bone.

_____ 7. The type of bone tissue filling the end of the long bone is called the:
   A. diaphysis.
   B. epiphysis.
   C. metaphysis.
   D. cancellous bone.
   E. compact bone.

_____ 8. The covering of the shaft of the long bones that initiates the bone repair cycle is the:
   A. periosteum.
   B. peritoneum.
   C. perforating canal.
   D. osteocyte.
   E. epiphysis.

_____ 9. Immovable joints such as those of the skull are termed:
   A. synovial.
   B. synarthroses.
   C. amphiarthroses.
   D. diarthroses.
   E. A or D

_____ 10. The smooth, flexible structures that act as the actual articular surface of joints are the:
   A. bursae.
   B. tendons.
   C. ligaments.
   D. cartilages.
   E. synovials.

_____ 11. The elbow is an example of which type of joint?
   A. monaxial
   B. biaxial
   C. triaxial
   D. synarthrosis
   E. amphiarthrosis

_____ 12. Bands of strong material that stretch and hold the joint together while permitting movement are the:
   A. bursae.
   B. tendons.
   C. ligaments.
   D. cartilage.
   E. metaphyses.

_____ 13. The small sacs filled with synovial fluid that reduce friction and absorb shock are the:
   A. bursae.
   B. tendons.
   C. ligaments.
   D. cartilage.
   E. metaphyses.

_____ 14. The most commonly fractured bone in the body is the:
   A. femur.
   B. pelvis.
   C. clavicle.
   D. humerus.
   E. scapula.

_____ 15. Which of the following is a bone of the upper arm?
   A. humerus
   B. radius
   C. olecranon
   D. phalanges
   E. carpal

_____ 16. Which of the following is a bone of the palm of the hand?
   A. humerus
   B. radius
   C. olecranon
   D. phalanges
   E. carpal

_____ 17. Which of the following is the bone of the thigh?
   A. tarsal
   B. tibia
   C. fibula
   D. femur
   E. phalanges

_____ 18. Skeletal maturity is reached by age:
   A. 6.
   B. 10.
   C. 20.
   D. 40.
   E. 45.

_____ 19. The muscular system consists of about how many muscle groups?
   A. 100
   B. 200
   C. 300
   D. 500
   E. 600

_____ 20. The muscle attachment to the bone that moves when the muscle mass contracts is the:
   A. flexor.
   B. extensor.
   C. origin.
   D. insertion.
   E. articulation.

_____ 21. More than half the energy created by muscle motion is in the form of heat energy.
   A. True
   B. False

_____ 22. Contusion can account for significant fluid loss into the more massive muscles of the body.
   A. True
   B. False

_____ 23. A specific sign associated with compartment syndrome is:
   A. deep pain.
   B. absent distal pulses.
   C. pain on passive extension.
   D. absent distal sensation.
   E. diaphoresis.

_____ 24. The condition in which exercise draws down the supply of oxygen and energy reserves and metabolic waste products accumulate, limiting the ability of a muscle group to perform is called:
   A. cramp.
   B. fatigue.
   C. strain.
   D. sprain.
   E. spasm.

_____ 25. The tissue that is normally damaged in a sprain is the:
   A. tendon.
   B. ligament.
   C. muscle.
   D. articular cartilage.
   E. epiphyseal plate.

_____ 26. The overstretching of a muscle that presents with pain is a:
   A. strain.
   B. sprain.
   C. cramp.
   D. spasm.
   E. subluxation.

_____ 27. Which of the following fractures is relatively stable?
   A. hairline
   B. impacted
   C. transverse
   D. comminuted
   E. both A and B

_____ 28. Which of the following fractures is most likely to be open?
   A. fibula
   B. tibia
   C. femur
   D. humerus
   E. ulna

_____ 29. In serious long bone fractures, especially those that are manipulated after injury, there is the possibility of fat embolizing and becoming lodged in the lungs.
   A. True
   B. False

_____ 30. Which of the following types of fractures is likely to occur only in the pediatric patient?
   A. greenstick
   B. oblique
   C. transverse
   D. comminuted
   E. spiral

_____ 31. The bones of the elderly are likely to be:
   A. less flexible.
   B. more brittle.
   C. more easily fractured.
   D. more slow to heal.
   E. all of the above

_____ 32. The dislocation, or fracture in the area of a joint, is generally less significant than the long bone shaft fracture because it does not have as high an incidence of vascular and nervous injury.
   A. True
   B. False

_____ 33. The energy and degree of manipulation needed to cause further injury after a bone has broken is much less than was initially needed to cause the fracture.
   A. True
   B. False

_____ 34. The growth of bone that comes after a fracture and encapsulates the fracture site is called the:
   A. epiphyseal outgrowth.
   B. periosteum.
   C. callus.
   D. natural splinting.
   E. comminution.

_____ 35. Which of the following is caused by a build-up of uric acid crystals in the joints?
   A. gout
   B. rheumatoid arthritis
   C. osteoarthritis
   D. bursitis
   E. tendinitis

_____ 36. An inflammation of the small synovial sacs that reduce friction and cushion tendons from trauma is:
   A. gout.
   B. rheumatoid arthritis.
   C. osteoarthritis.
   D. bursitis.
   E. tendinitis.

_____ 37. Which of the following is an indication for the use of PASG in the patient with skeletal injury?
   A. pelvic fracture
   B. serious tibial fracture
   C. femur fracture
   D. hip dislocation
   E. both A and D

_____ 38. With which of the fractures below should you consider immediate transport of the patient because of possible internal blood loss?
   A. humerus
   B. femur
   C. tibia
   D. pelvis
   E. both B and D

_____ 39. When assessing a limb for possible fracture, you should examine distally for:
   A. sensation.
   B. motor strength.
   C. circulation.
   D. crepitus.
   E. all of the above

_____ 40. A patient complains of a "pins and needles" sensation between the webs of his toes and a serious crushing-type injury has caused his calf to feel "almost board hard." What injury would you suspect?
   A. tibial fracture
   B. muscular contusion
   C. compartment syndrome
   D. tendinitis
   E. subluxation

_____ **41.** An elderly patient who has suffered a fracture due to bone degeneration is expected to experience what level of pain when compared to a traumatic fracture?
A. about the same
B. more pain
C. less pain
D. no pain at all
E. extreme pain

_____ **42.** As the effects of the fight-or-flight response wear off, the symptoms of fracture will become less evident.
A. True
B. False

_____ **43.** It is essential to tell the patient that limb alignment will cause some increased pain, as this will help maintain his or her confidence in you.
A. True
B. False

_____ **44.** In general, long bone shaft fractures should be splinted:
A. aligned, except if resistance is experienced.
B. as found.
C. extended, except if resistance is experienced.
D. flexed, except if resistance is experienced.
E. none of the above

_____ **45.** Any fracture within 3 inches of the joint should be treated as a dislocation.
A. True
B. False

_____ **46.** Which of the following positions is ideal for the immobilization of most extremity injuries?
A. extended
B. flexed
C. hyperextended
D. hyperflexed
E. neutral

_____ **47.** Ascending to altitude in a helicopter will cause the pressure in the air splint to:
A. increase.
B. decrease.
C. remain the same.
D. become less uniform.
E. become more uniform.

_____ **48.** The traction splint is designed to splint which musculoskeletal injury?
A. knee dislocation
B. hip dislocation
C. pelvic fracture
D. femur fracture
E. all of the above

_____ **49.** Which of the following is a disadvantage of the vacuum splint when applying it to splint fractures?
A. It is difficult to apply.
B. It is bulky and heavy.
C. It shrinks during application.
D. It takes more than two rescuers to apply.
E. all of the above

_____ **50.** Align a seriously angulated long bone fracture unless:
A. there is an absent distal pulse.
B. there is absent sensation.
C. both sensation and pulses are intact.
D. you meet with resistance.
E. you feel crepitus.

_____ **51.** If after moving a limb to alignment you notice the distal pulse is absent, you should:
A. splint the limb, as is.
B. gently move the limb to restore the pulse.
C. return the limb to the original positioning.
D. elevate the limb and then splint it.
E. splint and apply an ice pack.

_____ 52. With joint injury you should not move the limb around, even to restore circulation or sensation.
A. True
B. False

_____ 53. Early reduction of a dislocation usually results in which of the following?
A. less stress on the ligaments
B. less stress on the joint structure
C. better distal circulation
D. better distal sensation
E. all of the above

_____ 54. Signs that a reduction of a dislocation has been effective include:
A. feeling a "pop."
B. patient reports of less pain.
C. greater mobility in the joint.
D. less deformity of the joint.
E. all of the above

_____ 55. Heat may be applied to a muscular injury:
A. immediately.
B. after 1 hour.
C. after 24 hours.
D. after 48 hours.
E. not at all.

_____ 56. The splinting device recommended for a painful and isolated fracture of the femur is:
A. the vacuum splint.
B. the PASG.
C. the spine board and padding.
D. long padded board splints.
E. none of the above

_____ 57. The splinting device recommended for a painful and isolated fracture of the tibia is the:
A. traction splint.
B. PASG.
C. long spine board and padding.
D. padded board splint.
E. sling and swathe.

_____ 58. The splinting device recommended for an isolated fracture of the humerus is the:
A. traction splint.
B. sling and swathe.
C. air splint.
D. padded board splint.
E. both B and D

_____ 59. The fracture of the forearm close to the wrist that presents with the "silver fork" deformity is called:
A. Richardson's fracture.
B. Colles's fracture.
C. Volkman's contracture.
D. Blundot's inversion.
E. none of the above

_____ 60. An anterior hip dislocation normally presents with the:
A. foot turned outward.
B. foot turned inward.
C. knee flexed.
D. knee turned outward.
E. knee turned inward.

_____ 61. In general, anterior dislocations of the knee can be reduced in the prehospital setting.
A. True
B. False

_____ 62. Which of the following is NOT a sign of patellar dislocation?
A. knee in the flexed position
B. significant joint deformity
C. the extremity drops at the knee
D. lateral displacement of the patella
E. none of the above

_____ 63. If a patient presents with an ankle deformed with the foot turned to the side, you would suspect which type of ankle dislocation?
A. anterior
B. posterior
C. lateral
D. medial
E. inferior

_____ 64. If a patient presents with an ankle deformed with the foot pointing upward, you should suspect which type of ankle dislocation?
A. anterior
B. posterior
C. lateral
D. medial
E. inferior

_____ 65. When a patient's shoulder appears "squared-off," the patient complains of severe pain, and she cannot move her arm, you should suspect what type of shoulder dislocation?
A. anterior
B. inferior
C. superior
D. posterior
E. lateral

_____ 66. The elbow dislocation is a simple injury but one that it is essential to reduce in the field.
A. True
B. False

_____ 67. Which of the following injuries can be adequately splinted by using the short padded board splint, placing the hand in the position of function, and slinging and swathing the extremity?
A. radial fractures
B. ulnar fractures
C. wrist fractures
D. finger fractures
E. all of the above

_____ 68. Nitrous oxide in the prehospital setting:
A. is non-explosive.
B. reduces the perception of pain.
C. can be self-administered.
D. diffuses easily into air-filled spaces.
E. all of the above

_____ 69. Which of the following is NOT an analgesic that is used to control the pain of musculoskeletal injuries?
A. meperidine
B. morphine
C. nalbuphine
D. diazepam
E. none of the above

_____ 70. The "I" within acronym RICE used by athletic trainers stands for:
A. immobilization.
B. ice for the first 48 hours.
C. instability.
D. intensity of pain.
E. both A and B

SPECIAL PROJECTS

Recognizing Bones and Bone Injuries

I. Write the names of the bones marked with letters on the accompanying diagram of the human skeleton.

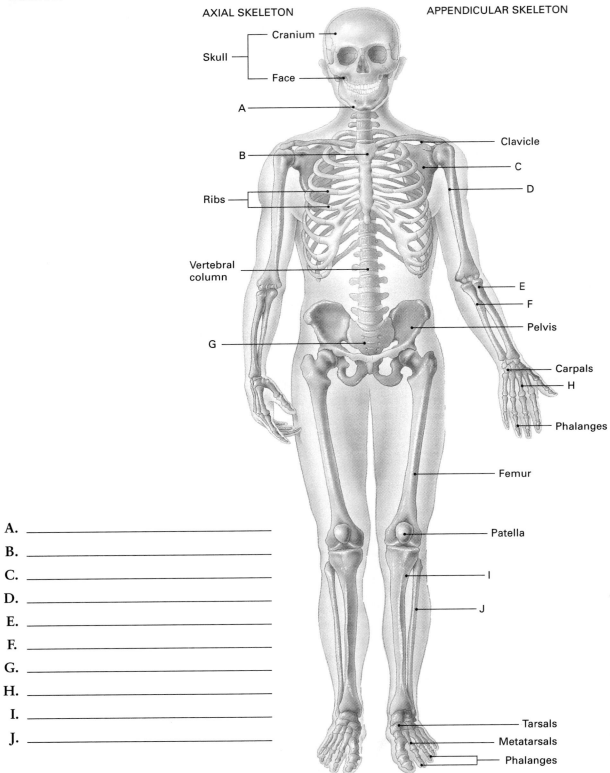

AXIAL SKELETON   APPENDICULAR SKELETON

Cranium

Skull

Face

A

Clavicle

B

C

Ribs

D

Vertebral column

E

F

Pelvis

G

Carpals

H

Phalanges

Femur

Patella

I

J

Tarsals

Metatarsals

Phalanges

A. _____

B. _____

C. _____

D. _____

E. _____

F. _____

G. _____

H. _____

I. _____

J. _____

II. Write the names of the types of fractures illustrated in the accompanying pictures.

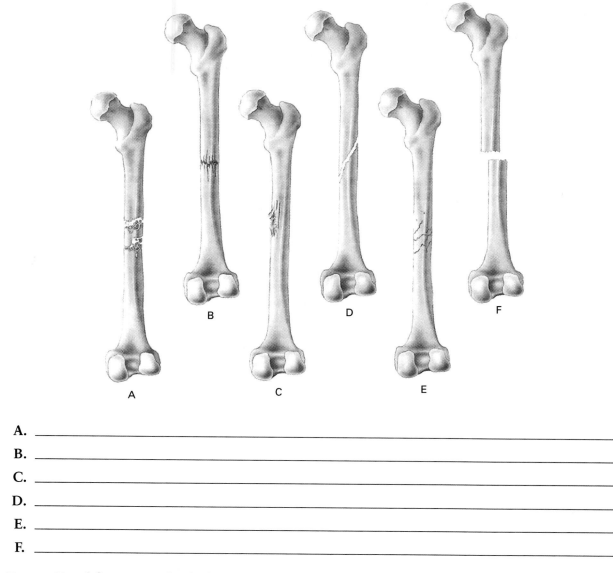

A. _____

B. _____

C. _____

D. _____

E. _____

F. _____

Drugs Used for Musculoskeletal Injuries

Emergency management for musculoskeletal injuries utilizes many of the pharmacologic agents that are available to the paramedic. Please review and memorize the various names/class, descriptions, indications, contraindications, precautions, dosages/routes for the following, with special attention to those used in your system. Use the drug flash cards found at the back of the Workbook for Volume 1.

Nitrous oxide

Diazepam

Morphine

Meperidine

Nalbuphine

CHAPTER 8

*

Head, Facial, and Neck Trauma

Review of Chapter Objectives

After reading this chapter, you should be able to:

1. Describe the incidence, morbidity, and mortality of head, facial, and neck injures.   **p. 263**

Approximately 4 million people experience significant head trauma each year, with 1 in 10 requiring hospitalization. Head trauma is the most common cause of trauma death, being especially lethal in auto collisions. Gunshot wounds to the head are less frequent but have a mortality of 75 to 80 percent. The population most at risk for head injury is the male between 15 and 24 years of age, infants and young children, and the elderly.

2. Explain the head and facial anatomy and physiology as they relate to head and facial injuries.   **pp. 263–276**

Several layers of soft, connective, and skeletal tissues protect the brain. These include the scalp, the cranium, and the meninges. The scalp is a thick and vascular layer of tissue that is strong and flexible and able to absorb tremendous kinetic energy. Beneath it are several layers of connective and muscular fascia that further protect the skull and its contents and that are only connected to the skull on a limited basis. This permits the scalp to move with glancing blows and further protect the cranium.

    The skull consists of numerous bones, fused together at fixed joints called sutures. These bones form a container for the brain called the cranium. The cranium is made up of three layers of bone, two thin layers of compact bone separated by a layer of cancellous bone. This construction makes the cranium both light and very strong. This vault for the brain is fixed in volume and does not accommodate any expansion of its contents. However, in the newborn and infant, the skull is more cartilaginous and more flexible, with two open areas, the anterior and posterior fontanelles. These spaces close by 18 months.

    The meninges are three layers of tissue—the dura mater, the arachnoid, and the pia mater—that provide further protection for the brain. The dura mater is a tough, fibrous layer that lines the interior of the skull and spinal foramen and is continuous with the inner periosteum of the cranium. The pia mater is a delicate membrane covering the convolutions of the brain and spinal cord. The arachnoid is a web-like structure between the dura mater and pia mater. The cerebrospinal fluid fills the subarachnoid space and "floats" the brain and spinal cord to help absorb the energy of trauma.

    The brain occupies about 80 percent of the volume of the cranium and is made up of the cerebrum, cerebellum, and brainstem. The cerebrum occupies most of the cranial vault and is the center of consciousness, personality, speech, motor control, and perception. It is separated into right and left hemispheres by the falx cerebri, extending inward from the anterior, superior, and posterior central skull. The cerebellum sits beneath the posterior half of the cerebrum and is responsible for fine tuning muscular control and for balance and muscle tone. It is separated from the cerebrum by the tentorium cerebelli, a fibrous sheath that runs transverse to the falx cerebri along the base of the cerebrum. The brainstem runs anterior to the cerebellum and central and inferior to the cerebrum. It consists of the hypothalamus, thalamus, pons, and medulla oblongata. The brainstem controls the endocrine system and most primary body functions including respiration, cardiac activity, temperature, and blood pressure.

The face, consisting of several bones covered with soft tissue, protects the special sense organs of sight, smell, hearing, balance, and taste and forms and protects the upper airway and the beginning of the alimentary canal. The brow ridge (a portion of the frontal bone), the nasal bones, and the zygoma form the eye sockets and protect the eyes. The upper jaw (the maxilla) and the moveable lower jaw (mandible) provide the skeletal structures that form the opening of the mouth. Cavities within this region (sinuses) help to provide shape to the face without increasing the weight of the head. The nasal cavity provides an extended surface to warm, humidify, and cleanse incoming air. The oral cavity houses the tongue and teeth and accommodates the early physical and chemical breakdown of food.

3. Predict head, facial, and other related injuries based on mechanism of injury.   **pp. 276–278**

Injuries to the head, face, and neck occur secondary to blunt or penetrating mechanisms. The most common cause of serious and blunt head trauma is the auto collision; other common mechanisms include falls, acts of violence, and, occasionally, sport-related activities. The neck is well protected both anteriorly and laterally, but it still may be impacted as the neck strikes the steering wheel or when the shoulder strap alone restrains movement of a vehicle's occupant. Penetrating injury is not as common as blunt injury but can still endanger life. Penetrating injuries to the cranium can be devastating to the brain tissue and are frequently not survivable, especially those injuries caused by high-energy gunshot wounds. Gunshot wounds to the face can also be life threatening as they may compromise the airway and distort facial and airway features.

4. Differentiate between the following types of facial injuries, highlighting the defining characteristics of each:

a. Eye   **pp. 273–275**

The eye is a globe filled with a crystal-clear fluid (vitreous humor) that focuses light through a lens onto light sensitive tissue, the retina. The amount of light entering the eye is determined by the size of the opening, the pupil (as controlled by the iris). The delicate surface of the eye is covered by the cornea (over the pupil and iris) and the conjunctiva (over the white portion of the eyeball, called the sclera). The eye is well protected from most blunt trauma by the skeletal structures of the brow ridge, zygomatic arch, and nasal bones. Blunt trauma may induce hyphema (blood filling the anterior chamber), subconjunctival hemorrhage (a blood-red discoloration of the sclera), and retinal detachment. Penetrating trauma or severe blunt trauma may directly injure the eye or entrap the small muscles that control it.

b. Ear   **pp. 272–273**

The external portion of the ear is the pinna, a cartilaginous structure covered by skin and only minimally supplied with circulation. A natural opening into the skull, the external auditory canal channels sound to the tympanum, where it and then the ossicles (the three bones of hearing) are set in motion. The ossicles vibrate the window of the cochlea, stimulating this organ of hearing to send impulses to the brain. The inner ear also houses the semicircular canals, which serve as an organ sensing head movement and balance. The pinna is easily injured, bleeds minimally, and heals poorly. Injury to the internal structures of the ear occurs very infrequently but may be caused by pressure differentials as with the blast over-pressures of an explosion, with the unequalized pressure associated with diving, or with direct insertion of an object into the ear canal.

c. Nose   **p. 272**

The nasal cavity is a pair of hollows formed by the junctures of the ethmoid, nasal, and maxillary bones. The external openings of the nose are the nares, formed by the nasal cartilage and anterior soft tissues. Frontal impact may fracture the nasal cartilage or bones, and severe Le Fort–type fractures may disrupt the nasal region. Since the area has a significant blood supply to warm incoming air, hemorrhage (epistaxis) can be heavy.

d. Throat
pp. 275–276

The throat or pharynx may be injured with lower facial or upper neck injury through either blunt or penetrating mechanisms. This region is made up of predominantly soft tissue and gains some support from the structure of the jaw and hyoid bones. Injury may fracture these bones, reducing the structural integrity of the region, or may damage soft tissues, resulting in massive swelling that threatens the airway. Any serious injury to this region is likely to endanger the airway.

e. Mouth
pp. 271–272

The mouth, or oral cavity, is made up of the upper and lower jaws, the hard and soft palates (superiorly), and the musculature and connective tissue in the base of the tongue. Fracture of the mandible and, to a lesser degree, the maxilla may reduce the structural integrity of the cavity and endanger its patency as a part of the airway. Injury may also result in severe soft-tissue swelling, hemorrhage, and in some cases, the loss of teeth.

5. Differentiate between facial injuries based on the assessment and history. pp. 289–294

The greatest dangers from skeletal or soft-tissue injury to the face are related to endangering of the airway, injury to the sensory organs housed and protected there, and damage to the cosmetic appearances of the region. The region is also very vascular and prone to serious blood loss. Facial fractures are classified according to the Le Fort criteria, with Le Fort I fractures relating to simple maxillary fractures, Le Fort II to fractures extending into the nasal bones, and Le Fort III to fractures involving the facial region all the way up to the brow ridge. These fractures are usually due to serious blunt trauma.

6. Explain the pathophysiology, assessment, and management for patients with eye, ear, nose, throat, and mouth injuries. pp. 289–302, 303–317

Eye injury may be due to blunt trauma and includes hyphema (blood in the eye's anterior chamber), conjunctival hemorrhage, or retinal detachment (the patient complaining of a curtain across part of the field of view). Severe blunt injury may cause orbital fracture, making it appear as though the eye was avulsed, or may entrap the ocular muscles and limit eye movement. Management includes covering both eyes with a cup over any protruding tissue or impaled object and bandaging. The patient must also be calmed and reassured because these injuries are very anxiety provoking. Penetrating eye trauma not only injures the delicate ocular tissue but also risks the loss of either aqueous or vitreous humors.

Ear injury most commonly affects the pinna and is due to glancing blows. Infrequently the internal organs of hearing and balance are damaged due to objects inserted into the ear or from dramatic pressure changes caused by explosions or diving injuries. External injury is cared for with dressing and bandaging, while with any internal injury the ear is covered with gauze to permit the drainage of any fluids from the external auditory canal.

Nasal injury can involve the nasal cartilage and bones and cause fractures or dislocations. Hemorrhage in this area (epistaxis) can be very heavy. If possible, the patient's head should be brought forward to ensure that blood from the nasal cavity drains outward and not down the throat, which could irritate the stomach and increase the likelihood of vomiting.

Injuries to the oral cavity are related to fractures of the mandible and associated soft-tissue destruction. Penetrating trauma, especially that produced by high-speed projectiles, can cause severe injury to the structures and tissues of the facial region and result in serious hemorrhage and danger to the patency of the airway. The airway should be maintained with suctioning, oral or nasal airway insertion, or with rapid sequence intubation, if necessary.

Pharyngeal injury is associated with serious risk of soft-tissue swelling and airway compromise. Use suction to remove fluids and consider early intubation because progressive swelling will restrict the airway and make later attempts at intubation more difficult.

7. Explain anatomy and relate physiology of the CNS to head injuries. pp. 264–269

The brain occupies 80 percent of the volume of the cranial vault. The brain consists of three major components: the cerebrum, the cerebellum, and the brainstem. The cerebrum is the center for conscious thought, perception, and motor control and is the largest structure within the cranium. The cerebellum fine tunes muscle movement and is responsible for muscle tone. The brainstem is made up of the thalamus, the hypothalamus, the pons, and the medulla oblongata. It is responsible for control of the vital signs and for consciousness. The central nervous system tissue is very delicate, very dependent upon adequate perfusion and a constant supply of oxygen, glucose, and thiamine, and easily injured by the forces of trauma. The contents of the cranium are protected by the scalp, the cranium, and the meninges. They are bathed in cerebrospinal fluid that floats them in a near-weightless environment.

8. Distinguish between facial, head, and brain injury.   pp. 278–295

Facial injury involves the soft or skeletal structures of the face, including the facial bones and mandible, the nasal cavity, the oral cavity, and the soft tissues covering the region. Their injury threatens the airway and the patient's cosmetic appearance. Serious facial injury is also suggestive of head and brain injury.

Head injury suggests that serious blunt or penetrating forces were expressed to the head with the potential for intracranial injury. Head injury involves damage to the scalp or cranium. It may also include brain (or intracranial) injury.

Brain injury is injury to the cerebrum, cerebellum, or brainstem. It may be caused by blunt trauma, either injuring tissue and blood vessels at the point of impact (coup injury) or injuring tissue and blood vessels away from the point of impact (contrecoup injury). Injury may also occur with an expanding lesion, as with epidural or subdural hematoma, with extensive cerebral edema that causes an increase in intracranial pressure, with a decrease in intracranial perfusion, and possibly with physical brain damage from pressure and displacement secondary to hemorrhage or edema.

9. Explain the pathophysiology of head/brain injuries.   pp. 276–295

Brain injury either is direct, related to the initial insult, or indirect, related to progressive pathologies secondary to the insult such as developing tissue irritation, inflammation, edema, hemorrhage, and physical displacement or by hypoxia. Direct injuries can be either coup or contrecoup in origin and include both the focal and diffuse injuries.

Focal injuries include cerebral contusion, which produces confusion and some local swelling, and intracranial hemorrhage, which produces hemorrhage as an arterial vessel above the dura mater ruptures and leads to a quickly evolving accumulation of blood and pressure (epidural hematoma) or as a venous vessel beneath the arachnoid membrane ruptures and produces a more gradual hemorrhage and build-up of pressure (subdural hematoma). Hemorrhage may also occur within the tissue of the brain (intracerebral hemorrhage) leading to a small accumulation of blood and some associated irritation, edema, and increase in intracranial pressure.

Diffuse injuries include the concussion (a mild or moderate diffuse axonal injury) and moderate and severe axonal injuries. These injuries are common and, with increasing severity, increasingly impair neurologic function and decrease the potential for return to a neurologically intact state. Diffuse injuries contuse, tear, shear, or stretch the brain tissue and cause injury that is often distributed throughout the brain.

Indirect injuries result as pressure displaces, compresses, or restricts the blood flow to regions of the brain. This secondary-type injury may induce hypoxia or ischemia that damages brain cells, causing inflammation and resulting in edema and further increases in ICP.

10. Explain the concept of increasing intracranial pressure (ICP).   pp. 285–287

The cranium is a rigid container with a fixed volume. It is full and each of its contents (cerebrum, cerebellum, brainstem, cerebrospinal fluid, and blood) occupies a component of the volume. Within this container, there is a limited constant pressure, the intracranial pressure. This pressure rarely exceeds 10 mmHg and at such a low level does not restrict cerebral blood flow. However, if one of the cranial residents increases its volume (vascular, as with hematoma, or the cerebrum itself, as with edema), another resident will have to decrease its volume or a pressure increase will result. During increasing ICP, some of the venous blood will leave the cranium, and then some cerebrospinal fluid will move to the spinal cord. These compensatory mechanisms work rather well, but the volume they can compensate for is limited. If expansion continues, the pressure (ICP) begins to rise. As it does, the difference between the intracranial pressure (ICP) and the mean arterial pressure (MAP) falls. This is the pressure driving cerebral perfusion (cerebral perfusion pressure, CPP). If CPP drops below 50 mmHg, cerebral perfusion pressure is not adequate to perfuse the brain. The body will increase the blood pressure in an attempt to maintain cerebral perfusion (autoregulation), but this only increases the edema or hemorrhage in a progressively worsening cycle.

11. Explain the effect of increased and decreased carbon dioxide on ICP.   pp. 285–287

Increased carbon dioxide concentrations in the blood cause the cerebral arteries to dilate and thereby provide better circulation to the contents of the cranium. This, however, can increase the intracranial pressure and increase any damage occurring due to a pre-existing elevated intracranial pressure.

      Decreased carbon dioxide causes vasoconstriction in the cerebral arteries and limits blood flow to the brain. If the blood CO_2 levels are reduced excessively, this will seriously limit cerebral blood flow and cause further injury to the patient who is already suffering from reduced cerebral blood flow (as with increased intracranial pressure).

12. Define and explain the process involved with each of the levels of increasing ICP.   pp. 285–287

The damage caused by increasing intracranial pressure (ICP) is progressive and limits cerebral perfusion. Normal intracranial pressure is very minimal and does not interfere with perfusion. However, as an injury (edema or an accumulation of blood) expands, it compresses the contents of the cranium. This compresses the veins and forces some venous blood from the cranium. If the pressure continues to rise, the pressure begins to move cerebrospinal fluid from the cranium (and into the spinal cord). If the pressure rise continues, arteries are compressed and cerebral blood flow suffers. This reduced circulation through the cerebrum causes a rise in the systemic blood pressure (autoregulation). This increases the cerebral blood flow but also increases the rate of intracranial hemorrhage and further increases the ICP. The result is a rapid rise in ICP, a reduction in cerebral blood flow, and cerebral hypoxia.

13. Relate assessment findings associated with head/brain injuries to the pathophysiologic process.   pp. 278–295

The most noticeable findings of brain injury are associated with the vital signs and include increasing blood pressure, erratic respirations (Cheyne-Stokes, Kussmaul's, central neurologic hyperventilation, or ataxic respirations), and a slowing pulse. These things are known collectively as Cushing's reflex. These signs indicate severe injury to the medulla oblongata, possibly due to its herniation into the foramen magnum. Eye signs, such as one pupil dilating and becoming unresponsive, are due to pressure on the oculomotor nerve as it is compressed against the tentorium. Such a sign is usually related to injury on the same (ipsilateral) side. The patient frequently demonstrates a reduced level of orientation or responsiveness and a Glasgow Coma Scale score of less than 15. The patient may also display retrograde or anterograde amnesia. These are generalized signs related to either diffuse axonal injury or increased intracranial pressure.

14. Classify head injuries (mild, moderate, severe) according to assessment findings.   pp. 296–303

Head injuries are classified according to the Glasgow Coma Scale. Those patients who score from 13 to 15 are considered to have received a mild injury, those from 9 to 12, a moderate injury, and those with a score of 8 or below are considered to have a severe head injury. Any change in the level of consciousness or orientation or any personality changes are signs of at least a mild head injury. Any finding that suggests the pulse rate is slowing, the respirations are becoming more erratic, and the blood pressure is rising due to head injury should be considered to indicate that the patient has a severe injury. The patient with the signs of a mild or moderate head injury must be watched very carefully because these pathologies frequently progress to more severe injuries.

15. **Identify the need for rapid intervention and transport of the patient with a head/brain injury.**　　pp. 296, 300–303

The pathologic processes at work in the patient with serious head injury are completely internal and cannot be repaired or stabilized in the field. High-flow oxygen administration and adequate ventilation (not hyperventilation) will ensure the best cerebral oxygenation without blowing off too much CO_2. Assuring good cardiovascular function and maintaining blood pressure are essential. In some systems, medications are also used to reduce cerebral edema in the field. However, often the only definitive way to correct the problems affecting the patient with serious head trauma is surgical intervention. For this reason, care for head injury patients focuses on bringing them quickly to a center capable of neurosurgical intervention.

16. **Describe and explain the general management of the head/brain injury patient, including pharmacological and nonpharmacological treatment.**　　pp. 303–315

The general management of the patient with recognized or suspected head injury begins with immobilization of the cervical spine to ensure no aggravation of any spinal injury. This manual immobilization is maintained and augmented by the application of a cervical collar, until the immobilization is continued by mechanical immobilization with a vest-type device or long spine board. The airway and adequate ventilation must be ensured. High-flow oxygen is the first-line drug for the patient with suspected head injury and complements ventilation to ensure the patient has good respirations, full breaths at 12 to 20 times per minute, without hyperventilation. Intubation may be attempted early using rapid sequence intubation with vecuronium as the paralytic of choice because succinylcholine may cause an increase in intracranial pressure. Mannitol may be beneficial as it draws fluid from the tissue with its osmotic properties and may reduce cerebral edema. Sedatives are indicated to premedicate the patient for the RSI procedure. Atropine will reduce airway secretions and may also reduce vagal stimulation and any increase in intracranial pressure that would otherwise occur during intubation attempts.

17. **Analyze the relationship between carbon dioxide concentration in the blood and management of the airway in the head/brain injured patient.**　　pp. 285–286, 308–309

In general, the higher the level of carbon dioxide in the blood, the greater the need to ventilate the patient. However, very low levels of carbon dioxide cause cerebral vasodilation, which may lead to a more rapidly increasing intracranial pressure. The objective of airway and respiratory care for the head injury patient is to assure a patent airway and good respiratory exchange without blowing off too much CO_2. This generally means that a patient should be ventilated with full breaths up to 20 times per minute.

18. **Explain the pathophysiology, assessment, and management of a patient with:**

   a. **Scalp injury**　　p. 315
   Scalp injuries tend to bleed heavily because their blood vessels do not constrict as well as those elsewhere on the body. This type of hemorrhage is easy to control because of the firm skull beneath, except when skull fracture is suspected. In that case, use distal pressure points and controlled direct pressure to stop any serious bleeding. Glancing injuries may expose the skull and flap the scalp over on itself. Remove any gross contaminants and cover the exposed surfaces with a sterile dressing. These injuries will heal very well due to the more than adequate blood supply they receive.

   b. **Skull fracture**　　pp. 298–299
   Skull fractures are skeletal injuries that usually heal uneventfully. The greatest concern is for the possible damage within the cranium. Skull fracture is anticipated by the mechanism of injury and should be suspected if fluids are draining out of the nose or ears. The retroauricular or bilateral periorbital ecchymoses associated with basilar skull fracture are not frequently seen in the prehospital setting because they take hours to develop. Immobilize the potentially fractured skull carefully and cover the ears and nose with gauze to assure free outward movement of any cerebrospinal fluid.

c. Cerebral contusion pp. 282, 295–315

The cerebral contusion is usually due to direct head trauma and may be the result of coup or contrecoup injury mechanisms. The patient may experience regional related neurologic deficits that resolve with time. This patient should be suspected of severe but more slowly progressive injury and watched very carefully. Administer oxygen and transport quickly.

d. Intracranial hemorrhage (including epidural, subdural, subarachnoid, and intracerebral hemorrhage) pp. 282–284, 287–288, 295–315

Intracranial hemorrhage (be it epidural, subdural, subarachnoid [a subset of subdural], or intracerebral) is a progressive injury mechanism that occurs as blood accumulates, displaces brain tissue, and raises intracranial pressure or as bleeding irritates brain tissue, initiates an inflammatory response, and causes cerebral edema and an increase in intracranial pressure. Patients with intracranial hemorrhage will display progressively deteriorating levels of orientation and consciousness and a history of serious head trauma. The elderly and chronic alcoholics may have an increased incidence of brain injury due to a reduced cerebral mass and more room for the brain to move during head trauma. Intracranial hemorrhage management includes oxygen, airway management, ensuring adequate ventilation, ensuring adequate blood pressure, and rapid transport. Rapid sequence intubation may be necessary, and mannitol may relieve some of the edema associated with the injury and ease the increased intracranial pressure.

e. Axonal injury (including concussion and moderate and severe diffuse axonal injury) pp. 284, 287–288, 295–315

Diffuse axonal injury may be anticipated by the mechanism of injury and by observation of any signs of progressively deteriorating levels of orientation and consciousness. Care is directed at oxygen administration, airway management, ensuring adequate ventilation, ensuring adequate blood pressure, and rapid transport. In severe cases, rapid sequence intubation may be necessary, and mannitol may relieve some of the edema associated with the injury and ease the increased intracranial pressure.

f. Facial injury pp. 289–294, 295–317

Facial injury may be anticipated by the mechanism of injury or recognized by soft-tissue injuries to or structural deformities of the region. Care is directed at maintaining the airway, protecting the eyes, and controlling any significant blood loss.

g. Neck injury pp. 294–295, 295–317

Neck injury is anticipated by the mechanism of injury and by a quick evaluation of the region. The spine is immobilized manually, a cervical collar is applied, and eventually manual immobilization is replaced with the mechanical immobilization of the vest-type immobilization device or the long spine board. Open soft-tissue injuries are covered with sterile dressings (or occlusive dressings if the injury is significant) and the airway is assessed to ensure that it is not at risk.

19. Develop a management plan for the removal of a helmet for a head-injured patient. p. 297

A helmet is carefully removed using techniques that limit the movement of the cervical spine and head. Full-face helmets provide the greatest challenge to removal, and to deal with them you should employ the techniques described in Chapter 9, "Spinal Trauma," of this text.

20. Differentiate between the types of head/brain injuries based on the assessment and history. pp. 276–303

The pathologies of head injury will either make your patient get progressively worse or better. Contusion and mild diffuse axonal injuries are likely to improve with time. However, as diffuse axonal injury gets more severe, the chances for recovery lessen and associated edema will likely increase the ICP and cause progressive neurologic deficit. Patients with intracranial hemorrhage (epidural and subdural) and intracerebral hemorrhage are likely to deteriorate with time. Epidural hemorrhage patients will show decreasing levels of consciousness and then the signs of increasing intracranial hemorrhage (eye signs, increasing systolic blood pressure, slowing and strengthening pulse, and erratic respirations). Patients with subdural and intracerebral hemorrhage will take longer to display these signs and may not do so in the prehospital setting. Be advised however, that one injury may be superimposed upon another. The concussion may render a patient unconscious and permit him to awaken, experience a lucid interval, and then deteriorate due to a developing epidural hematoma.

21. **Given several preprogrammed and moulaged head and facial injury patients, provide the appropriate scene size-up, initial assessment, focused assessment, detailed assessment, and then provide appropriate patient care and transportation.** pp. 295–317

During your training as an EMT-Paramedic you will participate in many classroom practice sessions involving simulated patients. You will also spend some time in the emergency departments of local hospitals as well as in advanced level ambulances gaining clinical experience. During these times, use your knowledge of head, facial, and neck trauma to help you assess and care for the simulated or real patients you attend.

CASE STUDY REVIEW

Reread the case study on pages 262 and 263 in Paramedic Care: Trauma Emergencies *before reading the discussion below.*

This case study presentation addresses the considerations of CNS injury in the auto accident. It looks at the elements of scene size-up, patient assessment, care, and transport, all with regard to the patient with potential head and spine injury.

The paramedics of unit 765 are dispatched to a typical auto collision with one patient. As Jan and Steve arrive at the scene, they note that the mechanism of injury is a frontal impact auto crash with severe vehicle deformity. This suggests that the patient is a candidate for rapid transport to the trauma center (trauma triage criteria). They also know that the crumple zones for frontal impact are extensive and vehicle deformity may somewhat spare occupant injury. Their analysis of the mechanism of injury notes a single star-shaped break in the windshield, suggesting an unrestrained driver and a potential for serious head injury. The driver's door ajar might suggest ejection and an increase in the suspected patient injuries. Jan and Steve anticipate head, chest, and lower extremity fractures from their analysis of the mechanism of injury.

Before the medics approach the vehicle they are careful to rule out scene hazards. They look for downed power lines, leaking gas or other fluid, any source of ignition for fire, traffic, jagged metal, and broken glass. They will also don gloves and have goggles, masks, and disposable gowns ready, just in case the danger of body fluid contamination should merit their use. They also ensure that the fire department is on-scene to stabilize the auto and to be ready in case there is any suggestion of fire danger. The police officer's report of the patient's unconsciousness supports the probability of head injury and the need for rapid transport.

As the medics arrive at the distorted auto, Jan immediately immobilizes John's head in a neutral position, facing directly forward, while Steve explains this is just a precaution and that he and Jan are paramedics there to aid John. During the initial assessment Steve determines John's mental status and finds he is somewhat disoriented to time and event. He remains disoriented even though Steve explains what time it is and that John was in an auto collision. This, coupled with the history of unconsciousness, clearly establishes a neurological problem, most likely associated with a head injury. They will move quickly to transport John to a neurocenter, if available, and will use the results of their initial neurologic assessment to trend any increase or decrease in John's orientation and level of consciousness. The airway appears fine as John is conscious, somewhat alert, and able to speak without encumbrance. Breathing is also adequate, but the patient's complaint of chest pain requires an investigation of the chest and reveals likely rib fractures, which may be limiting respiratory excursion and suggestive of pulmonary contusion underneath. Jan and Steve will frequently monitor breath sounds throughout their care to note any early development of pulmonary edema. They also attach ECG electrodes to monitor the heart in case of any myocardial contusion. Circulation appears very adequate with a strong pulse, good capillary refill, and a high oximetry reading. Nevertheless, Jan and Steve will constantly monitor the patient's signs and symptoms for any indication of the early development of shock.

Monitoring of the vital signs and level of consciousness may give evidence of progressing intracranial hemorrhage. An increase in blood pressure, reduction in pulse rate, erratic respirations, or decrease in orientation or level of consciousness would support the diagnosis. These signs and any other neurologic deficits will be documented and relayed to Medical Control to help identify the location of the injury and its progression.

Questioning by the paramedics during the initial assessment reveals a patient who cannot remember the events of the accident. This is a relatively common response, called retrograde amnesia. It is normal and by itself reflects a psychological response rather than a physiologic injury. As time progresses, the patient may begin to remember the accident. The patient questioning also investigates any medical history (the AMPLE elements of the medical history) or other condition that could have been a cause of the collision.

As the assessment continues, John becomes less alert, then unconscious (responding in a non-purposeful way to painful stimuli), and his left pupil dilates. These findings suggest increasing intracranial pressure, a serious condition that can only be corrected at a neurocenter. As the patient begins to deteriorate, Jan and Steve employ rapid extrication techniques to move him to the long spine board. He is secured quickly, and the crew begins transport is to the neurocenter. Once John is unconscious and is no longer able to control his airway, Steve intubates him and assures full breaths at 16 per minute. While hyperventilation might increase oxygenation, it might also blow off excessive carbon dioxide, constrict cerebral arteries, and further reduce blood flow to the brain. Steve places the endotracheal tube quickly to reduce the increase in intracranial pressure caused by vagal stimulation during intubation attempts. He may use a topical anesthetic spray like xylocaine or benzocaine to reduce vagal stimulation or premedicate with atropine to prevent a vagal response and possible dysrhythmias.

CONTENT SELF-EVALUATION

MULTIPLE CHOICE

_____ 1. The most common cause of trauma-related death is due to injury to the:
   A. head.
   B. thorax.
   C. abdomen.
   D. pelvis.
   E. extremities.

_____ 2. What percentage of penetrating wounds to the cranium result in mortality?
   A. 30 to 40 percent
   B. 40 to 50 percent
   C. 65 to 70 percent
   D. 75 to 80 percent
   E. 90 to 95 percent

_____ 3. Which of the following is a layer of the scalp?
   A. the skin
   B. occipitalis muscle
   C. galea aponeurotica
   D. areolar tissue
   E. all of the above

_____ 4. Which of the following is NOT a bone of the cranium?
   A. frontal
   B. mandible
   C. parietal
   D. sphenoid
   E. ethmoid

_____ 5. The largest opening in the cranium is the:
   A. auditory canal.
   B. orbit of the eye.
   C. foramen magnum.
   D. tentorium.
   E. transverse foramen.

_____ 6. Place the following layers of the meninges as they occur from the cerebrum to the skull.
   A. dura mater, pia mater, arachnoid
   B. dura mater, arachnoid, pia mater
   C. arachnoid, pia mater, dura mater
   D. arachnoid, dura mater, pia mater
   E. pia mater, arachnoid, dura mater

_____ 7. The layer of the meninges that is strong and lines the interior of the cranium is the:
   A. pia mater.   D. dura mater.
   B. falx cerebri.   E. tentorium.
   C. arachnoid.

_____ 8. The structure that divides the cerebrum into left and right halves is the:
   A. pia mater.   D. dura mater.
   B. falx cerebri.   E. tentorium.
   C. arachnoid.

_____ 9. The cerebellum is the center of conscious thought and perception.
   A. True
   B. False

_____ 10. Which of the following is a function of the hypothalamus?
   A. body temperature control
   B. control of the ascending reticular activating system
   C. control of respiration
   D. responsiblity for sleeping
   E. maintaining balance

_____ 11. Which of the following is a function of the thalamus?
   A. body temperature control
   B. control of the ascending reticular activating system
   C. control of respiration
   D. responsiblity for sleeping
   E. maintaining balance

_____ 12. Which of the following is a function of the medulla oblongata?
   A. body temperature control
   B. control of the ascending reticular activating system
   C. control of respiration
   D. responsiblity for sleeping
   E. maintaining balance

_____ 13. While the brain accounts for only 2 percent of the total body weight, it requires 15 percent of the cardiac output and 20 percent of the body's oxygen supply.
   A. True
   B. False

_____ 14. The capillaries serving the brain are thicker and less permeable than those in the rest of the body.
   A. True
   B. False

_____ 15. The normal intracranial pressure is:
   A. 120 mmHg.   D. 25 mmHg.
   B. 90 mmHg.   E. less than 10 mmHg.
   C. 50 mmHg.

_____ 16. The reflex that increases the systemic blood pressure to maintain cerebral blood flow is called:
   A. the ascending reticular activating system.
   B. the descending reticular activating system.
   C. autoregulation.
   D. Cushing's reflex.
   E. mean arterial pressure.

_____ 17. Which of the following nerves is responsible for slowing the heart rate?
   A. CN-I   D. CN-X
   B. CN-III   E. CN-XII
   C. CN-VIII

_____ 18. Which of the following nerves is responsible for voluntary movement of the tongue?
  A. CN-I
  B. CN-III
  C. CN-VIII
  D. CN-X
  E. CN-XII

_____ 19. Which of the following is the lower and movable jaw bone?
  A. the maxilla
  B. the mandible
  C. the zygoma
  D. the stapes
  E. the pinna

_____ 20. Which of the following is the bone of the cheek?
  A. the maxilla
  B. the mandible
  C. the zygoma
  D. the stapes
  E. the pinna

_____ 21. The structure responsible for our positional sense is the:
  A. ossicle.
  B. cochlea.
  C. semicircular canals.
  D. sinuses.
  E. vitreous humor.

_____ 22. Which of the following is the opening through which light travels to contact the light-sensing tissue in the eye?
  A. retina
  B. aqueous humor
  C. vitreous humor
  D. pupil
  E. iris

_____ 23. Which of the following is the light-sensing tissue in the eye?
  A. retina
  B. aqueous humor
  C. vitreous humor
  D. pupil
  E. iris

_____ 24. The white of the eye is the:
  A. sclera.
  B. conjunctiva.
  C. cornea.
  D. aqueous humor.
  E. vitreous humor.

_____ 25. The delicate, clear tissue covering the pupil and iris is the:
  A. sclera.
  B. conjunctiva.
  C. cornea.
  D. aqueous humor.
  E. vitreous humor.

_____ 26. Which of the following nerves control eye movement?
  A. CN-II
  B. CN-III
  C. CN-IV
  D. CN-VI
  E. all except A

_____ 27. Head trauma accounts for about what percentage of motor vehicle–related deaths?
  A. 20 percent
  B. 40 percent
  C. 50 percent
  D. 80 percent
  E. 90 percent

_____ 28. Serious scalp injury is unlikely to produce hypovolemia and shock as the arteries there frequently constrict and effectively limit blood loss.
  A. True
  B. False

_____ 29. Which of the following statements is NOT true of scalp wounds?
  A. They pose a risk of meningeal infection.
  B. Wounds there tend to heal very well.
  C. Wounds there tend to bleed heavily.
  D. Contusions there swell outward noticeably.
  E. Avulsion of the scalp is not a likely injury.

_____ 30. The most common type of skull fracture is:
   A. depressed.
   B. basilar.
   C. linear.
   D. comminuted.
   E. spiral.

_____ 31. The type of skull fracture most often associated with high-velocity bullet entry is:
   A. depressed.
   B. basilar.
   C. linear.
   D. comminuted.
   E. spiral.

_____ 32. It is common for the paramedic to observe either Battle's sign or bilateral periorbital ecchymosis in the patient who has just sustained a basilar skull fracture.
   A. True
   B. False

_____ 33. The discoloration found around both eyes due to basilar skull fracture is:
   A. retroauricular ecchymosis.
   B. bilateral periorbital ecchymosis.
   C. Cullen's sign.
   D. the halo sign.
   E. Gray's sign.

_____ 34. Blood and CSF draining from the ear may display a:
   A. speckled appearance.
   B. concentric lighter yellow circle.
   C. congealed mass.
   D. greenish discoloration.
   E. none of the above

_____ 35. A cranial fracture, by itself, is a skeletal injury that will heal with time; it is the injury underneath that is of most concern.
   A. True
   B. False

_____ 36. The type of injury that causes damage to the brain on the side opposite the impact is called:
   A. coup.
   B. subdural hematoma.
   C. subluxation.
   D. contrecoup.
   E. concussion.

_____ 37. Which of the following is considered a focal injury?
   A. cerebral contusion
   B. epidural hematoma
   C. subdural hematoma
   D. intracerebral hemorrhage
   E. all of the above

_____ 38. Which of the following injuries is most likely to cause the patient to deteriorate rapidly?
   A. cerebral contusion
   B. epidural hematoma
   C. subdural hematoma
   D. intracerebral hemorrhage
   E. concussion

_____ 39. Which of the following is an injury with venous bleeding into the arachnoid space?
   A. cerebral contusion
   B. epidural hematoma
   C. subdural hematoma
   D. intracerebral hemorrhage
   E. concussion

_____ 40. The injury that classically presents with unconsciousness immediately after the accident followed by a lucid interval and then a decreasing level of consciousness is most likely a(n):
   A. concussion.
   B. epidural hematoma.
   C. subdural hematoma.
   D. cerebral hemorrhage.
   E. both A and B

_____ 41. Which of the following head injuries would you NOT expect to get worse with time?
   A. intracerebral hemorrhage
   B. subdural hematoma
   C. concussion
   D. epidural hematoma
   E. intracranial hemorrhage

_____ 42. Indirect brain injury occurs as a result of, but after, initial injury.
   A. True
   B. False

_____ 43. As intracranial hemorrhage begins, it first displaces which occupant of the cranium?
   A. cerebrospinal fluid
   B. venous blood
   C. arterial blood
   D. oxygen
   E. the pia matter

_____ 44. Perfusion through the cerebrum is a factor of intracranial pressure and:
   A. systolic blood pressure.
   B. diastolic blood pressure.
   C. mean arterial pressure.
   D. cerebral perfusion pressure.
   E. none of the above

_____ 45. High levels of carbon dioxide in the blood will cause which of the following?
   A. hyperventilation
   B. cerebral artery constriction
   C. cerebral artery dilation
   D. hypertension
   E. none of the above

_____ 46. Vomiting, changes in the level of consciousness, and pupillary dilation result from herniation of the upper brainstem through the:
   A. tentorium incisura.
   B. foramen magnum.
   C. falx cerebri.
   D. transverse sinus.
   E. tentorium cerebelli.

_____ 47. Cushing's reflex includes which of the following?
   A. erratic respirations
   B. increasing blood pressure
   C. slowing heart rate
   D. A and B
   E. A, B, and C

_____ 48. Which of the following respiratory patterns is NOT indicative of brain injury?
   A. eupnea
   B. ataxic respirations
   C. central neurogenic hyperventilation
   D. Cheyne-Stokes respirations
   E. agonal respirations

_____ 49. In the presence of intracranial pressure, the fontanelles of the infant will:
   A. withdraw.
   B. become stiff.
   C. bulge.
   D. pulsate.
   E. atrophy.

_____ 50. Increasing intracranial pressure is likely to cause pupillary dilation on the ipsilateral side.
   A. True
   B. False

_____ 51. With facial trauma, airway obstruction is more likely due to blood than other fluids or physical obstruction.
   A. True
   B. False

_____ 52. According to the Le Fort criteria, a fracture involving just the maxilla and limited instability is classified as:
   A. Le Fort I.
   B. Le Fort II.
   C. Le Fort III.
   D. Le Fort IV.
   E. Le Fort V.

_____ 53. Which type of Le Fort fracture is likely to result in cerebrospinal fluid leakage?
   A. Le Fort I
   B. Le Fort II
   C. Le Fort III
   D. Le Fort IV
   E. Le Fort V

_____ 54. Which of the following statements is TRUE regarding injuries to the pinna of the ear?
A. They hemorrhage severely.
B. Hemorrhage is difficult to control.
C. Hemorrhage is limited.
D. Wounds there do not heal very well.
E. both C and D

_____ 55. Which of the following mechanisms is likely to injure the tympanum?
A. basilar skull fracture
B. an explosion
C. diving injury
D. an object forced into the ear
E. all of the above

_____ 56. The collection of blood in front of a patient's pupil and iris due to blunt trauma is called a(n):
A. hyphema.
B. retinal detachment.
C. aniscoria.
D. anterior chamber hematoma.
E. sub-conjunctival hemorrhage.

_____ 57. A sudden and painless loss of sight is most likely a(n):
A. hyphema.
B. retinal detachment.
C. acute retinal artery occlusion.
D. anterior chamber hematoma.
E. sub-conjunctival hemorrhage.

_____ 58. Blood vessel injury in the neck region carries with it the hazards of all of the following EXCEPT:
A. severe venous hemorrhage.
B. severe arterial hemorrhage.
C. development of subcutaneous emphysema.
D. air aspiration.
E. pulmonary emboli.

_____ 59. The patient with a suspected brain injury should be ventilated with full breaths:
A. 8 to 10 times per minute.
B. 12 to 20 times per minute.
C. 20 to 24 times per minute.
D. 24 to 30 times per minute.
E. 30 to 36 times per minute.

_____ 60. Which of the following is a probable sign of increasing intracranial pressure?
A. decreasing pulse strength
B. weakening pulse strength
C. slowing pulse rate
D. increasing pulse strength
E. both C and D

_____ 61. The major reason for allowing fluid to drain from the nose or ear is that:
A. it may slow the rise of intracranial pressure
B. its flow will prevent pathogens from entering the meninges
C. it is impossible to stop the flow anyway
D. regeneration of CSF is beneficial to the healing process
E. none of the above

_____ 62. When light intensity changes in one eye and both respond, this response is called:
A. diplopia.
B. aniscoria.
C. consensual reactivity.
D. synergism.
E. photophobia.

_____ 63. Any significant open wound to the anterior or lateral neck should be covered with a(n):
A. wet dressing.
B. occlusive dressing.
C. nonadherent dressing.
D. adherent dressing.
E. pressure dressing.

_____ 64. When a patient reports of sensitivity to light, this is an example of:
A. diplopia.
B. aniscoria.
C. consensual reactivity.
D. synergism.
E. photophobia.

_____ 65. During your assessment you determine that the patient exhibits confused speech, follows simple commands, and opens his eyes on his own. What Glasgow Coma Scale value would you assign?

A. 15
B. 14
C. 12

D. 10
E. 7

_____ 66. The highest Glasgow Coma score is:

A. 20.
B. 15.
C. 12.

D. D+.
E. a score that varies with each patient.

_____ 67. A patient who responds only to pain and then only flexes, mutters incomprehensible words when shouted at loudly, and opens his eyes only to pain is given what Glasgow Coma Scale score?

A. 14
B. 12
C. 10

D. 8
E. 6

_____ 68. Which of the following could be considered a component of Cushing's reflex?

A. Cheyne-Stokes respirations
B. decreasing pulse rate
C. increasing blood pressure

D. ataxic respirations
E. all of the above

_____ 69. The head injury patient may vomit without warning and the vomiting may be projectile in nature.

A. True
B. False

_____ 70. If the head injury patient is found without any other suspected injuries, what positioning would be best for her?

A. the Trendelenburg position
B. with the head of the spine board elevated 30 degrees
C. left lateral recumbent position
D. immobilized completely and rolled to her side
E. none of the above

_____ 71. Which of the following airway techniques is NOT acceptable for the patient with suspected basilar skull fracture?

A. nasopharyngeal airway insertion
B. directed intubation
C. digital intubation

D. orotracheal intubation
E. rapid sequence intubation

_____ 72. The process of inserting an endotracheal tube increases the intracranial pressure and should only be done by the care provider most experienced in the procedure.

A. True
B. False

_____ 73. Which of the following is an acceptable method for confirming endotracheal tube placement in the head injury patient?

A. use of an end-tidal CO_2 monitor
B. use of a pulse oximeter
C. observing bilaterally equal chest rise
D. good and bilaterally equal breath sounds
E. all of the above

_____ 74. For adequate ventilation through a needle cricothyrotomy, you must use a demand valve ventilator.

A. True
B. False

_____ 75. When locating the cricoid cartilage, either for Sellick's maneuver or the cricothyrotomy, it is the first hard rigid ring you feel as you move your fingers up the trachea from the suprasternal notch.
   A. True
   B. False

_____ 76. Ventilation of the head injury patient should be guided by oximetry to maintain a saturation of at least:
   A. 80 percent.   D. 95 percent.
   B. 85 percent.   E. 98 percent.
   C. 90 percent.

_____ 77. Care for the patient with increasing intracranial pressure must NOT include aggressive fluid resuscitation, even if the patient's blood pressure drops below 60 mmHg.
   A. True
   B. False

_____ 78. In the head injury patient you must keep the blood pressure above:
   A. 50 mmHg.   D. 120 mmHg.
   B. 60 mmHg.   E. none of the above
   C. 90 mmHg.

_____ 79. Which of the following drugs is the first-line diuretic in the treatment of head injury?
   A. oxygen   D. succinylcholine
   B. mannitol   E. morphine
   C. furosemide

_____ 80. Which of the following paralytics increases ICP and should be used with caution, if at all, in head injury patients?
   A. diazepam   D. succinylcholine
   B. mannitol   E. midazolam
   C. vecuronium

_____ 81. It is recommended to administer diazepam by adding it first to the plastic IV bag as this assures a uniform administration.
   A. True
   B. False

_____ 82. Which of the following drugs will reverse the effects of diazepam and midazolam?
   A. narcan   D. thiamine
   B. flumazenil   E. none of the above
   C. atropine

_____ 83. Which of the following actions of atropine make it a desirable adjunct to rapid sequence intubation?
   A. It reduces vagal stimulation.
   B. It reduces airway secretions.
   C. It reduces fasciculations.
   D. It helps maintain heart rate during intubation.
   E. all of the above

_____ 84. Dextrose is administered to the head injury patient:
   A. routinely.   D. for suspected diabetes or alcoholism.
   B. for hyperglycemia only.   E. with hetastarch.
   C. for hypoglycemia only.

_____ 85. Dislodged teeth from a patient should be:
   A. wrapped in gauze soaked in water.
   B. wrapped in gauze soaked in sterile saline.
   C. wrapped in dry gauze.
   D. kept dry but cool.
   E. replaced immediately.

SPECIAL PROJECT

Crossword Puzzle

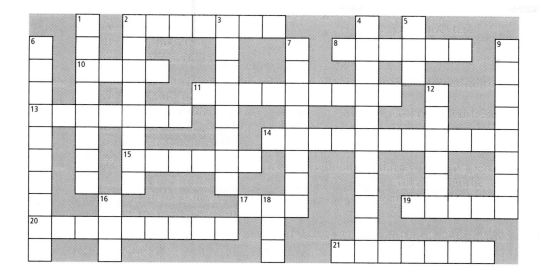

Across
2. Winding cone-shaped tube that is part of the inner ear
8. Light-sensitive lining of the inner eye
10. _____ mater; outermost of the meninges
11. _____ membrane; middle layer of the meninges
13. Falx _____ ; division of the cerebrum into right and left halves
14. _____ amnesia; inability to remember events after a trauma that caused the condition
15. Referring to the long communications pathways of nerve cells
17. Device used in mechanically immobilizing a patient (abbr.)
19. Openings of the nostrils
20. Medulla _____ ; lower portion of the brainstem
21. _____ Coma Scale; predictor of head injury severity

Down
1. Portion of the brain connecting the pons and cerebellum
2. Referring to the brain
3. _____ fluid; liquid that lubricates the eye
4. Bilateral _____ ecchymosis; black-and-blue discoloration around the eyes
5. _____ mater; innermost of the meninges
6. Mild or moderate form of diffuse axonal injury (DAI)
7. One of the bones making up the base of the skull
9. _____ humor; clear, watery fluid filling the posterior chamber of the eye
12. Thin, delicate layer covering the pupil and iris
16. A patient's mental acuity (abbr.)
18. Pressure exerted on the brain by the blood and the cerebrospinal fluid

Composing a Radio Message and Run Report

Preparing both the radio message to the receiving hospital and the written run report are two of the most important tasks you will perform as a paramedic. Reread the case study on pages 262 and 263 of Paramedic Care: Trauma Emergencies *and then read the additional information about the call provided below. From this information compose a radio message and complete the run report for this call.*

The Call

Dispatch to the call comes from the 911 Center at 2:15 AM. It directs Unit 765 to an auto accident at the junction of Highway 127 and Country Trunk H, in Wilbur Township. They arrive at the scene at 2:32 to find one male occupant of the vehicle who is 31 years old.

The initial care of the patient includes spinal immobilization (2:33), cervical collar (2:34), vitals, (2:36) and oxygen @ 10L via nonrebreather mask (2:36). A second set of vitals is taken just after the patient becomes unconsciousness. They reveal a pulse of 52, respirations of 22 deep and labored, blood pressure of 136/88, and a pulse oximeter reading of 98 percent. The patient is responsive to painful stimuli only (2:41). The patient is immobilized to a long spine board (2:41), loaded on the stretcher, and moved to the ambulance at 2:42 with transport begun immediately.

En route, an initial IV is started in the left forearm with a 16-gauge angiocatheter to run normal saline (1,000 mL) at a "to-keep-open" rate. You are headed to the Community Hospital, the closest facility and the base of your medical direction.

Medical Control is contacted and you call in the following:

The medical direction physician instructs you to bring your patient to the Medical Center and orders that an endotracheal tube be placed if possible. An 8.0 mm tube is positioned orally via digital technique with good bilateral breath sounds auscultated (2:51). The vitals are repeated (pulse, 62; BP, 142/92; respirations, 24 deep and irregular; pulse oximeter, 97%).

You contact Medical Control and provide the following update:

Your ETA to the Medical Center is now 15 minutes. The second set of vital signs taken en route show the following: BP, 140/90; pulse, 50 and bounding; respirations, 25 (assisted by BVM), and pulse oximetry of 97 percent (3:01). The patient is delivered to the Medical Center at 3:15, and you report for service at 3:55.

Complete the Prehospital Care Report on the next page from the information contained in the narrative of this call.

Date	Emergency Medical Services Run Report	Run # 913

Patient Information | Service Information | Times

Name:	Agency:	Rcvd :
Address:	Location:	Enrt :
City: St: Zip:	Call Origin:	Scne :
Age: Birth: / / Sex: [M][F]	Type: Emrg[ ] Non[ ] Trnsfr[ ]	LvSn :
Nature of Call:		ArHsp :
Chief Complaint:		InSv :

Description of Current Problem:

Medical Problems

Past		Present
[ ]	Cardiac	[ ]
[ ]	Stroke	[ ]
[ ]	Acute Abdomen	[ ]
[ ]	Diabetes	[ ]
[ ]	Psychiatric	[ ]
[ ]	Epilepsy	[ ]
[ ]	Drug/Alcohol	[ ]
[ ]	Poisoning	[ ]
[ ]	Allergy/Asthma	[ ]
[ ]	Syncope	[ ]
[ ]	Obstetrical	[ ]
[ ]	GYN	[ ]

Other:

Trauma Scr: Glasgow:

On Scene Care:	First Aid:
	By Whom?

02 @ L : Via	C-Collar :	S-Immob. :	Stretcher :

Allergies/Meds:	Past Med Hx:

Time	Pulse	Resp.	BP S/D	LOC	ECG
:	R: [r][i]	R: [s][l]	/	[a][v][p][u]	
Care/Comments:					
:	R: [r][i]	R: [s][l]	/	[a][v][p][u]	
Care/Comments:					
:	R: [r][i]	R: [s][l]	/	[a][v][p][u]	
Care/Comments:					
:	R: [r][i]	R: [s][l]	/	[a][v][p][u]	
Care/Comments:					

Destination:	Personnel:	Certification
Reason:[ ]pt [ ]Closest [ ]M.D. [ ]Other	1.	[P][E][O]
Contacted: [ ]Radio [ ]Tele [ ]Direct	2.	[P][E][O]
Ar Status: [ ]Better [ ]UnC [ ]Worse	3.	[P][E][O]

Now, compare the radio message and the run report form that you prepared against the examples in the Answer Key of this workbook. As you make this comparison, keep in mind that there are many "correct" ways to communicate this body of information. Ensure that you have recorded the major points of your assessment and care and enough other material to describe the patient and his condition to the receiving physician and anyone who might review the form. Remember that this document may be the only record of your assessment and care for this patient. When you are done, it should be a complete accounting of your actions.

Drugs Used for Head, Facial, and Neck Injuries

Emergency management for head injury utilizes many of the pharmacologic agents that are available to the paramedic. Please review and memorize the various names/class, descriptions, indications, contraindications, precautions, and dosages/routes for the following, with special attention to those used in your system. Use the drug flash cards found at the back of the workbook for Volume 1.

Mannitol	Midazolam
Furosemide	Morphine
Succinylcholine	Atropine
Pancuronium	Dextrose
Vecuronium	Thiamine
Diazepam	

CHAPTER 9
*
Spinal Trauma

Review of Chapter Objectives

After reading this chapter, you should be able to:

1. Describe the incidence, morbidity, and mortality of spinal injuries in the trauma patient. pp. 322–323

Spinal cord injuries account for over 15,000 permanent injuries, occurring most frequently in males aged from 16 to 30. Auto collisions account for almost half of the injuries, while falls, penetrating injuries, and sports-related injuries also contribute significantly to the toll. Spinal cord injuries are especially devastating because they affect the very specialized tissue of the central nervous system, which has relatively little ability to repair itself, and because the cord is the major communication conduit of the body. Injury often results in permanent loss of function below the lesion.

2. Describe the anatomy and physiology of structures related to spinal injuries, including:

a. Cervical spine pp. 323–326

The cervical spine is the vertebral column between the cranium and the thorax. It consists of seven irregular bones held firmly together by ligaments that both support the weight of the head and permit its motion while protecting the delicate spinal cord that runs through the central portion of these bones.

b. Thoracic spine pp. 323–327

The thoracic vertebral column consists of 12 thoracic vertebrae, one corresponding to each rib pair. Like the cervical spine, it consists of irregular bones held firmly together by ligaments that support the weight of the head and neck and permit its motion while protecting the delicate spinal cord that runs through the central portion of these bones.

c. Lumbar spine pp. 323–325, 327

The lumbar spine consists of five lumbar vertebrae with massive vertebral bodies to support the weight of the head, neck, and thorax. Here the spinal cord ends at the juncture between L-1 and L-2 and nerve roots fill the spinal foramen from L-2 into the sacral spine.

d. Sacrum pp. 323–325, 327

The sacrum consists of five sacral vertebrae that are fused into a single plate that forms the posterior portion of the pelvis. The upper body balances on the sacrum, which articulates with the pelvis at a fixed joint, the sacroiliac joint.

e. Coccyx pp. 323–325, 327

The coccygeal region of the spine consists of three to five fused vertebrae that form the remnant of a tail.

f. Spinal cord pp. 327–329

The spinal cord is a component of the central nervous system consisting of very specialized nervous system cells that do not repair themselves very well. The cord is the body's major communications conduit, sending motor commands to the body and returning sensory information to the brain.

g. **Nerve tracts**   pp. 329–333

The nerve tracts are pathways within the spinal cord for impulses from distinct areas and with distinct sensory or motor functions. The two major types of nerve tracts are ascending tracts, those that carry sensory information to the brain, and descending tracts, those that carry motor commands to the body.

h. **Dermatomes**   pp. 331–332

The dermatomes are distinct regions of the body's surface that are sensed by specific peripheral nerve roots. For example, the collar region is sensed by C3, the nipple line is sensed by T4, the umbilicus is sensed by T10, and the lateral (little) toe is sensed by S1. These landmarks are useful in denoting where the loss of sensation occurs, secondary to spinal injury.

3. Predict spinal injuries based on mechanism of injury.   pp. 333–336

Most spinal trauma is related to extremes of motion. These include extension/flexion, lateral bending, rotation, and axial loading/distraction. These types of movement place stresses on the vertebral column that stretch and injure the ligaments, fracture the vertebral elements, rupture the intervertebral disks, and dislocate the vertebra. While these are all connective or skeletal tissue injuries, they threaten the protective function served by the vertebral column and endanger the spinal cord. The injury mechanism itself or further movement of the vertebral column may cause the skeletal elements to compress, contuse, lacerate, sever, or stretch the cord, resulting in neurologic injury and a deficit below the level of injury.

A frontal impact injury mechanism is likely to cause axial loading and a crushing-type injury to the spine as well as flexion injury (as may occur in the auto or diving incidents). Lateral impact auto collisions are likely to cause lateral bending injury, while rear-end impacts are likely to cause extension, then flexion injury. Hangings may cause distraction injury. Rotational injuries may occur during sporting events.

Penetrating injury is a direct type of injury that disrupts the connective and skeletal structure of the vertebral column and may directly involve the spinal cord. Deep and powerful knife injuries and bullet wounds are the most common mechanisms of this injury.

4. Describe the pathophysiology of spinal injuries.   pp. 336–339

The spinal cord, like all central nervous system tissue, is extremely specialized and delicate and does not repair itself well, if at all. The spinal cord may be injured in much the same way as the brain by mechanisms including concussion, contusion, compression, laceration, hemorrhage, and transection. The concussion is a jarring that momentarily disrupts the cord function. Contusion results in some damage and bleeding into the cord but will likely repair itself. Compression may occur due to vertebral body displacement or as a result of cord edema; it deprives portions of the cord of blood, and ischemic damage may result. The degree of injury and its permanence is related to the amount of compression and the length of time the compression remains. Laceration occurs as bony fragments are driven into the cord and damage it. If the injury is severe, the injury is probably permanent. Hemorrhage into the cord results in compression and irritation of the cord tissue as blood crosses the blood-brain barrier. The injury may also restrict blood flow to a portion of the cord, extending the injury. Transection is a partial or complete severance of the cord with its function below the lesion, for the most part, lost.

5. Identify the need for rapid intervention and transport of the patient with spinal injuries.   pp. 322–323, 340–346

The need for rapid intervention and transport of the spinal injury patient must take into account the key element of prehospital care, which is immobilizing the vertebral column to restrict motion and any further injury. Once injured, the vertebral column can no longer protect the spinal cord from injury and, in fact, becomes the source of probable injury with manipulation. It is imperative that the head be brought to the neutral position and maintained there until the injury heals, it is corrected surgically, or X-rays and CT scans rule out injury. This means that once spinal injury is suspected, the patient remains immobilized until delivered to the emergency department.

6. Describe the pathophysiology of traumatic spinal injury related to:

- **Spinal shock**   **p. 338**

  Spinal shock is a transient form of neurogenic shock due to a temporary injury to the spinal cord. It results as the brain loses control over body functions including vasoconstriction, motor control, and sensory perception below the level of injury.

- **Spinal neurogenic shock**   **pp. 338–339**

  Neurogenic shock is a more permanent result of cord injury resulting in loss of control over body functions including vasoconstriction, motor control, and sensory perception below the level of injury. The injury results in an inability to control peripheral vascular resistance and blood pressure.

- **Quadriplegia/paraplegia**   **pp. 337–338**

  The loss of neurologic control over the lower extremities (paraplegia) and the loss of control over all four limbs (quadriplegia) is related to the location of the spinal cord lesion. The higher the injury along the vertebral column, the more of the body is affected. These injuries are related to the distribution of the dermatomes for sensation and myotomes for motor control. Injuries at or below the thoracic spine (T3) involve the lower extremities (paraplegia) while injuries above this level affect all four extremities (quadriplegia).

- **Incomplete and complete cord injury and cord syndromes**   **pp. 337–338**

  Injury to the spinal cord can result from the mechanisms discussed earlier. A complete cord injury completely severs the spinal cord, and the potential to send and receive nerve impulses below the site of the injury is lost. Results may include, depending on the site of injury, incontinence, paraplegia, quadriplegia, and partial or complete respiratory paralysis.

  With incomplete cord injury, the spinal cord is only partially severed. There is potential for recovery of function. There are three common types of incomplete cord syndrome:

- **—Central cord syndrome**   **p. 338**

  Central cord syndrome is related to hyperextension-type injuries and is often associated with a pre-existing disease like arthritis that narrows the spinal foramen. It usually results in motor weakness of the upper extremities and in some cases loss of bladder control. The prognosis for at least some recovery for the central cord syndrome is the best of all the cord syndromes.

- **—Anterior cord syndrome**   **p. 338**

  Anterior cord syndrome is due to damage caused by bone fragments or pressure on the arteries that perfuse the anterior portion of the cord. The affected limbs are likely only to retain motion, vibration, and positional sensation with motor and other perceptions lost.

- **—Brown-Séquard's syndrome**   **p. 338**

  Brown-Séquard's syndrome is most often caused by a penetrating injury that affects one side of the cord (hemitransection). Sensory and motor loss is noted on the ipsilateral side, while pain and temperature sensation is lost on the contralateral side. The injury is rare but often associated with some recovery.

7. Describe the assessment findings associated with and management for traumatic spinal injuries.   **pp. 340–362**

The primary assessment finding used to determine the need for spinal precautions is the mechanism of injury. Vertebral column injury may present with only minimal signs and symptoms of injury, often overshadowed by more painful injuries. Failure to immobilize the spine early during assessment and care may lead to vertebral column movement and damage to the spinal cord.

The signs and symptoms of spinal injury include pain or tenderness along the spinal column, any neurologic deficit, especially if it corresponds to the dermatomes and is bilateral, including any deficits in sensation to touch, temperature, motion, vibration, etc. Any loss in the ability to move (paralysis) or muscular strength (paresis) is suggestive of spinal cord injury. Special signs associated with spinal injury include an involuntary erection of the penis (priapism), loss of bowel and bladder control, and diaphragmatic breathing.

8. **Describe the various types of helmets and their purposes.**   p. 352

Helmets are made for use in contact sports, bicycling, skateboarding, in-line skating, and motor-cycling. Some helmets are partial and can be easily removed at the accident scene. Other helmets (football, for example) completely enclose the head and may be difficult to remove at the accident scene and may pose immobilization problems for prehospital care givers. It must be remembered that, while helmets offer some protection for the head, they have not been proven to reduce spinal injuries.

9. **Relate the priorities of care to factors determining the need for helmet removal in various field situations including sports-related incidents.**   p. 352

Remember that while a helmet provides some protection for head injury, it does not necessarily protect the spine. Take immobilization precautions if the mechanism of injury suggests the potential for spinal injury. If the patient can be fully immobilized with the helmet on, it can be left in place. However you must remove a helmet if the helmet does not immobilize the patient's head, if the helmet cannot be securely immobilized to the long spine board, if it prevents airway care, or if it prevents assessment of anticipated injuries. The helmet should also be removed if you anticipate development of airway or breathing problems. Always be sure that helmet removal will not cause further injuries.

    Procedures for helmet removal will vary with the type of helmet. The prime consideration is to continue to maintain manual immobilization of the patient throughout whatever procedure is used and then to assure that the patient receives proper mechanical immobilization once the helmet is removed.

10. **Given several preprogrammed and moulaged spinal injury patients, provide the appropriate scene size-up, initial assessment, rapid trauma assessment, detailed assessment, and then provide the appropriate patient care and transport.**   pp. 340–362

During your training as an EMT-Paramedic you will participate in many classroom practice sessions involving simulated patients. You will also spend some time in the emergency departments of local hospitals as well as in advanced-level ambulances gaining clinical experience. During these times, use your knowledge of spinal trauma to help you assess and care for the simulated or real patients you attend.

CASE STUDY REVIEW

Reread the case study on pages 321 and 322 in Paramedic Care: Trauma Emergencies *before reading the discussion below.*

    This case highlights the precautions that must be taken whenever there is a possibility of spinal injury.

Fred and Lisa respond to a blunt injury impact on the football field. They work with the team's athletic trainer and listen very carefully to his and the patient's description of the mechanism of injury as they begin their initial assessment. His torso was impacted from the side, probably displacing the chest laterally while the head and neck remained stationary. Either the impact caused the injury or injury was caused by the impact with the ground. As they begin their care for Bill, the paramedics don sterile gloves and form a general impression of Bill. He is an otherwise healthy young male who is able to speak in complete sentences and appears oriented to time, place, and persons. After a check of Bill's distal pulse, Fred and Lisa quickly rule out any serious and immediate threats to Bill's airway, breathing, and circulation.

    As Fred and Lisa move to the focused trauma exam, they investigate the complaint of "tingling" and assess the spine from the base of the head to the sacrum and then determine which dermatomes are affected by the paresthesia. They note tenderness around the 7th thoracic vertebra, a relatively common site for spine injury with lateral impact. The dermatomes affected are consistent with a lower cervical injury (most of the upper extremity is spared). With such conclusive evidence of a spinal column and cord injury, Fred and Lisa will be very careful in their helmet removal, movement of the patient to the long spine board, and spinal immobilization procedures. They will also carefully monitor for the signs and symptoms of neurogenic shock (warm lower limbs and cool upper limbs and the signs of hypovolemic compensation).

Fred and Lisa are presented with a dilemma regarding the helmet. It firmly immobilizes Bill's head within but due to its spherical nature it would be extremely difficult to affix to the flat surface of the long spine board. They choose to remove the helmet and secure Bill's head directly to the spine board. They are also very attentive to the proper positioning of Bill's head. Normally it would rest about 1 to 1½ inches above the posterior body plane. However, because of Bill's shoulder padding, to achieve proper positioning the head must be kept well above the playing field. They carefully remove the pads and lower the head, with the shoulders, to just slightly above the level of the field. They choose to use axial traction to move Bill to the long spine board as it will help keep the spine in alignment during the move and requires fewer participants. As they move and secure Bill to the spine board, they assure that the head rests the appropriate 1 to 1½ inches above the surface of the board.

In some Advanced Life Support systems, Bill may have received either methylprednisolone or dexamethasone for the suspected spinal cord injury. Its administration may be helpful in reducing inflammation and edema associated with the injury and hence the extent of injury.

During the entire procedure Lisa and Fred calm and reassure Bill that their actions are, for the most part, precautionary and explain each action before they perform it. This reduces Bill's anxiety. Clearly the proper spinal precautions, as performed by this paramedic team, were responsible for limiting the seriousness of Bill's injuries.

CONTENT SELF-EVALUATION

MULTIPLE CHOICE

_____ 1. The vertebral column is made up of how many vertebrae?
   A. 24
   B. 33
   C. 43
   D. 45
   E. 54

_____ 2. The major weight-bearing component of the vertebral column is the:
   A. spinous process.
   B. transverse process.
   C. vertebral body.
   D. spinal foramen.
   E. lamina.

_____ 3. The intravertebral disks account for what percentage of the spinal column's height?
   A. 10
   B. 25
   C. 30
   D. 40
   E. 50

_____ 4. The region of the vertebral column that has 12 vertebrae is the:
   A. cervical.
   B. thoracic.
   C. lumbar.
   D. sacral.
   E. coccygeal.

_____ 5. The region of the vertebral column that permits the greatest movement is the:
   A. cervical.
   B. thoracic.
   C. lumbar.
   D. sacral.
   E. coccygeal.

_____ 6. The region of the vertebral column that has five separate vertebrae is the:
   A. cervical.
   B. thoracic.
   C. lumbar.
   D. sacral.
   E. coccygeal.

_____ 7. The structure of the meninges of the spinal column is similar to the structure of the meninges of the cranium.
A. True
B. False

_____ 8. At its distal end, the spinal cord is attached to the:
A. foramen magnum.
B. peripheral nerve roots.
C. sacral ligament.
D. lumbar process.
E. coccygeal ligament.

_____ 9. The region of the spine with the closest tolerance between the spinal cord and the interior of the spinal foramen is the:
A. cervical spine.
B. thoracic spine.
C. lumbar spine.
D. sacral spine.
E. coccygeal spine.

_____ 10. The nerve tissues responsible for communicating sensory impulses to the brain is(are) the:
A. white matter.
B. gray matter.
C. ascending tracts.
D. descending tracts.
E. myotomes.

_____ 11. The nerve tissues consisting of nerve cell axons and making up the exterior portion of the spinal cord is(are) the:
A. white matter.
B. gray matter.
C. ascending tracts.
D. descending tracts.
E. myotomes.

_____ 12. The region of the spine that has one more pair of nerve roots than it does vertebrae is the:
A. cervical spine.
B. thoracic spine.
C. lumbar spine.
D. sacral spine.
E. coccygeal spine.

_____ 13. The S-1 nerve root controls the:
A. collar region.
B. little finger.
C. nipple line.
D. umbilicus.
E. small toe.

_____ 14. The T-10 nerve root controls the:
A. collar region.
B. little finger.
C. nipple line.
D. umbilicus.
E. small toe.

_____ 15. Which of the following motions is likely to result from the rear-end auto impact?
A. extension
B. flexion
C. lateral bending
D. axial loading
E. distraction

_____ 16. Which of the following motions is likely to result from hanging?
A. extension
B. flexion
C. lateral bending
D. axial loading
E. distraction

_____ 17. Spinal cord injury can occur without injury to the vertebral column or its associated ligaments.
A. True
B. False

_____ 18. The region that accounts for more than half of spinal cord injuries is the:
A. cervical spine.
B. thoracic spine.
C. lumbar spine.
D. sacral spine.
E. coccygeal spine.

_____ 19. A spinal cord concussion is likely to produce residual deficit.
   A. True
   B. False

_____ 20. The region of the vertebral column in which the spinal cord ends is the:
   A. cervical.   D. sacral.
   B. thoracic.   E. coccygeal.
   C. lumbar.

_____ 21. Spinal shock is a temporary form of neurogenic shock.
   A. True
   B. False

_____ 22. Which of the following is a sign associated with neurogenic shock?
   A. priapism
   B. decreased heart rate
   C. decreased peripheral vascular resistance
   D. warm skin below the injury
   E. all of the above

_____ 23. Which of the following is associated with the resolution of shock due to cord injury and results in hypertension?
   A. autonomic hyperreflexia syndrome
   B. neurogenic shock
   C. spinal shock
   D. central cord syndrome
   E. both B and D

_____ 24. Which of the following is NOT a mechanism of injury likely to cause spinal injury?
   A. fall from over three times the patient's height
   B. high-speed motor vehicle crash
   C. serious blunt trauma above the shoulders
   D. penetrating trauma directed to the lateral thorax
   E. penetrating trauma directed to the spine

_____ 25. Helmets reduce the incidence of both head and spine injury.
   A. True
   B. False

_____ 26. Oral intubation is generally more difficult in the patient who requires spinal precautions because the landmarks are more difficult to visualize.
   A. True
   B. False

_____ 27. During the initial assessment, you should be aware that exaggerated abdominal movement and limited chest excursions often suggest:
   A. airway obstruction.
   B. the need to reposition the head and neck.
   C. diaphragmatic breathing.
   D. neurogenic shock.
   E. cardiac contusion.

_____ 28. During your assessment of a patient, you find sensation is lost as you move from the lower extremities all the way up to the level of the collar. This is probably due to an injury at which spinal level?
   A. C-3   D. T-10
   B. T-1   E. S-1
   C. T-4

_____ 29. The "hold-up" positioning of the arms is due to injury at or around:
    A. C-3.   D. T-10.
    B. T-1.   E. S-1.
    C. T-4.

_____ 30. Which of the following is indicative of spinal injury?
    A. increased heart rate   D. a normal body temperature
    B. increasing blood pressure   E. none of the above
    C. excessive chest expansion

_____ 31. Proper immobilization of the patient with spinal injury should include placing a blanket roll under the knees.
    A. True
    B. False

_____ 32. The most ideal position for the adult head during spinal immobilization is:
    A. 1 to 2 inches above the spine board
    B. level with the spine board
    C. with padding under the shoulders and the head on the spine board
    D. with the head slightly extended and level with the board
    E. none of the above

_____ 33. Which of the following is a contraindication to continuing to move the head and spine toward the neutral, in-line position?
    A. You meet with significant resistance.
    B. Your patient complains of a significant increase in pain.
    C. You notice gross deformity along the spine.
    D. You notice an increase in the signs of neurologic injury.
    E. all of the above

_____ 34. Some gentle axial traction on the head will make cervical immobilization more effective.
    A. True
    B. False

_____ 35. The ideal position for the small adult's or child's head during spinal immobilization is:
    A. 1 to 2 inches above the spine board
    B. level with the spine board
    C. with padding under the shoulders and the head on the spine board
    D. with the head slightly extended and level with the board
    E. none of the above

_____ 36. The standing takedown for the patient with spinal injuries requires a minimum of how many care providers?
    A. two   D. five
    B. three   E. no less than six
    C. four

_____ 37. Under which of the following circumstances should a helmet be removed from a patient?
    A. The head is not immobilized within the helmet.
    B. The helmet prevents airway maintenance.
    C. You cannot secure the helmet firmly to the long spine board.
    D. You anticipate breathing problems.
    E. all of the above

_____ 38. A four-count cadence is preferable for moves as it better signals care providers when the move starts.
    A. True
    B. False

_____ **39.** Orthopedic stretchers are not rigid enough to be used for spinal immobilization by themselves.
   A. True
   B. False

_____ **40.** The vest-type immobilization device is meant to permit rescuers to move the patient from a seated to a supine position in an auto crash by rotating the buttocks on the seat, then tilting the patient to the supine position.
   A. True
   B. False

_____ **41.** Which of the following circumstances would not automatically merit employment of rapid extrication techniques?
   A. toxic fumes
   B. an auto collision
   C. an immediate threat of fire
   D. rising water
   E. none of the above

_____ **42.** Once you immobilize the body to the long spine board, you can then secure the head to it.
   A. True
   B. False

_____ **43.** Which of the following is used in the prehospital setting for the treatment of spine injuries?
   A. mannitol
   B. methylprednisolone
   C. dexamethasone
   D. furosemide
   E. both B and C

_____ **44.** If a suspected spinally injured patient does not respond to fluid resuscitation, which drug would you consider?
   A. methylprednisolone
   B. atropine
   C. furosemide
   D. dopamine
   E. diazepam

_____ **45.** To address bradycardia in the suspected spinally injured patient, which drug would you consider?
   A. methylprednisolone
   B. atropine
   C. furosemide
   D. dopamine
   E. diazepam

SPECIAL PROJECTS

Recognizing Spinal Regions

Label the regions of the spine and the number of the vertebrae in each.

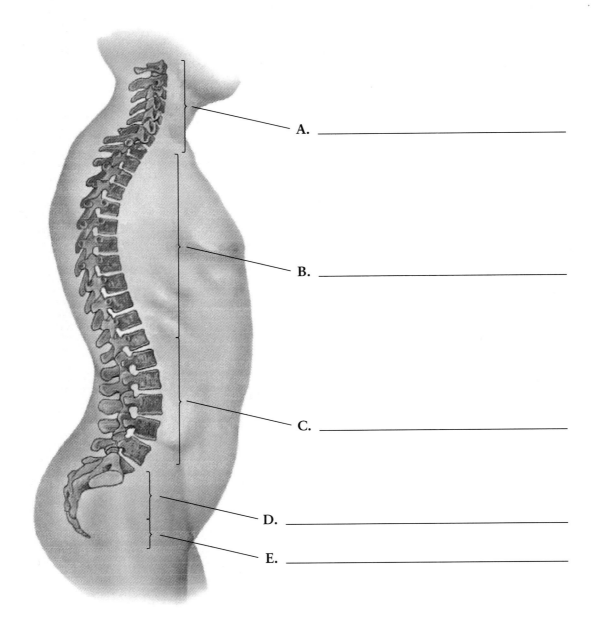

A. _____

B. _____

C. _____

D. _____

E. _____

Recognizing Dermatomes

In the spaces provided below, write in the areas of the body affected by each of the dermatomes indicated.

C-3 _____

T-1 _____

T-4 _____

T-10 _____

S-1 _____

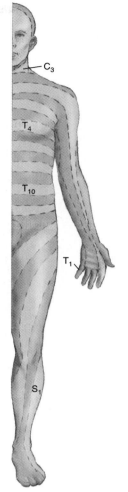

Drugs Used for Spinal Injuries

Emergency management for spinal injuries utilizes many of the pharmacologic agents that are available to the paramedic. Please review and memorize the various names/class, descriptions, indications, contraindications, precautions, and dosages/routes for the following, with special attention to those used in your system. Use the drug flash cards found at the back of the Workbook for Volume 1.

    Methylprednisolone

    Dexamethasone

    Dopamine

    Atropine

    Meperidine

    Diazepam

CHAPTER 10
Thoracic Trauma

Review of Chapter Objectives

After reading this chapter, you should be able to:

1. Describe the incidence, morbidity, and mortality of thoracic injuries in the trauma patient.

pp. 366–367

Chest trauma accounts for about 25 percent of vehicular mortality and is second only to head trauma as a reason for death in the auto accident. Heart and great vessel injuries are the most common cause of death from blunt trauma. Penetrating trauma to the chest also results in significant mortality with heart and great vessel injuries, again, accounting for the greatest mortality. Modern auto and highway design, the speed at which the chest trauma patient arrives at the trauma center, and newer surgical techniques have significantly reduced chest trauma mortality in the last decade.

2. Discuss the anatomy and physiology of the organs and structures related to thoracic injuries.

pp. 367–379

The ribs, thoracic spine, sternum, and diaphragm define the structure of the thoracic cage. The skeletal components allow the cage to expand as the ribs are lifted upward and outward by contraction of the intercostal muscles, and the intrathoracic volume further expands as the diaphragm contracts and moves downward. The net action of this muscle movement is to increase the volume of the thoracic cage and to reduce its internal pressure. Air from the environment moves through the airway into the alveoli to equalize this pressure, and inspiration occurs. The intercostal muscles relax and the thorax settles, while the diaphragm rises back into the thorax and the volume of the cavity decreases. This increases the intrathoracic pressure, and air rushes out to equalize with the environment. This is expiration. The pleura, two serous membranes, seal the lungs to the interior of the thoracic cage during this action and ensure that the lungs expand and contract with the changing volume of the thoracic cavity. The lungs have exceptional circulation, with capillary beds surrounding the alveoli to assure a free exchange of oxygen and carbon dioxide between the alveolar air and the bloodstream.

The lungs fill all but the central portion of the chest cavity and are found on either side of the central structure, called the mediastinum. The mediastinum contains the heart, trachea, esophagus, major blood vessels, and several nerve pathways. The heart is located in the left central chest and is the major pumping element of the cardiovascular system. The inferior and superior vena cavae collect blood from the lower extremities and abdomen and the upper extremities, head, and neck, respectively, and return it to the heart. The pulmonary arteries and veins carry blood to and from the lungs respectively, and the aorta distributes the cardiac output to the systemic circulation. The trachea enters the mediastinum just beneath the manubrium and bifurcates at the carina into the left and right mainstem bronchi. The esophagus enters the mediastinum just behind the trachea and exits through the diaphragm.

3. Predict thoracic injuries based on mechanism of injury.

pp. 380–382

As in other regions of the body, thoracic trauma results from either blunt or penetrating mechanisms of injury. Blunt trauma may result from deceleration (as in an auto crash), crushing mechanism (as in a building collapse), or pressure injury (as with an explosion). Deceleration frequently causes the "paper bag" syndrome, lung and cardiac contusions, rib fractures, and vascular injuries. Crushing mechanisms may cause traumatic asphyxia and vascular damage and restrict respiratory excursion. Blast mechanisms may cause lung injuries or vascular tears.

Penetrating trauma may involve any structure within the thorax, although injury to the heart and great vessels is most likely to be lethal. Lung tissue is rather resilient and suffers limited injury with a bullet's passage, while the heart and great vessels are damaged explosively, especially if engorged with blood at the time of the bullet's impact. Slower velocity penetrating objects result in damage that is limited to the actual pathway of the object.

4. Discuss the pathophysiology of, assessment findings with, and the management and need for rapid intervention and transport of the patient with chest wall injuries, including:

a. Rib fracture
pp. 383–385, 406

Blunt or penetrating trauma induces a fracture and possible associated injury underneath. The fracture itself is of only limited concern; however, the pain from an such injury may limit chest excursion and suggests more serious injury beneath. Care is directed to administering oxygen, considering the possibility of underlying injury, and supplying pain medication to assure respirations are not limited by pain. These injuries do not by themselves require immediate intervention or transport.

b. Flail segment
pp. 385–386, 406

A flail segment is the result of several ribs (three or more) broken in numerous (two or more) places. This creates a rib segment that is free to move independently from the rest of the thorax. This paradoxical motion greatly decreases the efficiency of respiration as air that would be exhaled moves to the region under the flail segment and then returns to the unaffected lung with inspiration. Care includes seeing that the section is stabilized, the patient is given oxygen, possibly using overdrive ventilation. Consider the flail chest patient a candidate for rapid transport. Because of the severity of forces required to compromise the chest wall with this injury and the likelihood of serious underlying injury, this patient is given a high priority for care and transport.

c. Sternal fracture
p. 385

As with the flail chest patient, suspect the patient with sternal fracture of having serious internal injury. The kinetic forces necessary to fracture the sternum are likely to injure and contuse the heart and other structures of the mediastinum. The patient will have a history of blunt chest trauma and may complain of chest pain similar to that of a myocardial infarction. Administer oxygen, monitor the heart with an ECG, and watch the patient very carefully for any signs of myocardial or great vessel injury. This patient is a candidate for rapid transport.

5. Discuss the pathophysiology of, assessment findings with, and management and need for rapid intervention and transport of the patient with injury to the lung, including:

a. Simple pneumothorax
pp. 378–388

A simple or closed pneumothorax is an injury caused by either blunt or penetrating trauma that opens the airway to the pleural space. Air accumulates within the space and displaces the lung, resulting in less effective respirations and reduced oxygenation of the blood. This patient has a history of trauma and progressive dyspnea. Oxygen is administered and the patient is observed for progression to tension pneumothorax.

b. Open pneumothorax
pp. 388–389, 407

Open pneumothorax is like simple pneumothorax, though in this case the injury penetrates the thoracic wall. The injury must be significantly large in order for air to move preferentially through the wound. The patient will have an open chest wound and dyspnea. Care includes sealing the wound on three sides to prevent further progress of the pneumothorax, provision of oxygen, and monitoring the patient for the development of tension pneumothorax.

c. Tension pneumothorax   pp. 389–390, 407–409

Tension pneumothorax is a pneumothorax created under the mechanisms associated with simple or open pneumothorax that progresses because of a valve-like injury site. The valve permits air to enter the pleural space but not exit. This results in a progressive lung collapse, followed by increasing pressure that displaces the mediastinum and restricts venous return to the heart. The patient has a trauma history and progressive dyspnea that becomes very severe. The patient may also display subcutaneous emphysema and distended jugular veins. Care is directed at decompressing the thorax with the insertion of a catheter into the 2nd intercostal space, providing oxygen, and monitoring the patient for a recurring tension pneumothorax.

d. Hemothorax   pp. 390–391, 409

A hemothorax is a collection of blood in the pleural space. It may occur with or without pneumothorax. Hemothorax will generally become a hypovolemic problem before it seriously endangers respiration because the amount of fluid loss necessary to restrict respiration is great. The patient may experience dyspnea and the signs and symptoms of hypovolemic compensation (shock). Provide the patient with shock care, oxygen, fluid replacement, and rapid transport.

e. Hemopneumothorax   p. 391

A hemopneumothorax is simply the existence of blood loss into the pleura and an accumulation of air there. Its presentation includes the signs and symptoms associated with both these pathologies. Care is directed at oxygen administration and rapid transport.

f. Pulmonary contusion   pp. 391–392

Pulmonary contusion is a blunt trauma injury to the tissue of the lung resulting in edema and stiffening of the lung tissue. This reduces the efficiency of air exchange and causes an increased workload associated with respiration. If the region involved is limited, the patient may only experience very mild dyspnea. If the area is extensive, the patient may experience severe dyspnea. Care is centered around assuring good oxygenation, including overdrive ventilation when indicated, and rapid transport.

6. Discuss the pathophysiology of, findings of assessment with, and management and need for rapid intervention and transport of the patient with myocardial injuries, including:

a. Myocardial contusion   pp. 393–394, 409

Myocardial contusion is simply a contusion to the myocardium, usually related to blunt anterior chest trauma. The patient will present with myocardial-infarction-like pain and possible dysrhythmias. Care is directed at oxygen therapy, cardiac medications as indicated, and rapid transport.

b. Pericardial tamponade   pp. 394–395, 409

Pericardial tamponade is usually related to penetrating trauma in which a wound permits blood from within the heart to enter the pericardium. It progressively fills the pericardium and restricts ventricular filling. The cardiac output drops and circulation is severely restricted. The patient will present with a penetrating trauma mechanism and will move quickly into shock, and possibly, sudden death. Care is insertion of a needle into the pericardial sac and the withdrawal of fluid. Any patient suspected of this injury requires immediate transport to the closest hospital.

c. Myocardial rupture   p. 395

Myocardial rupture is often associated with high-velocity penetrating trauma. The bullet's passage through the engorged heart causes the blood to move outward from the bullet's path (cavitation) explosively. The heart wall tears, and the patient hemorrhages extensively as cardiac output ceases. The patient will display the signs of sudden death and no resuscitation efforts will be successful.

7. **Discuss the pathophysiology of, findings of assessment with, and management and need for rapid intervention and transport of the patient with vascular injuries, including injuries to:**

a. **Aorta**   **pp. 396, 409**

Aortic aneurysm is a ballooning of the aorta as blunt trauma shears open the tunica intima and tunica media. Blood under systolic pressure enters the injury site and begins to dissect the vessel, causing it to balloon like a tire's inner tube. The patient will have a history of blunt trauma and complain of a tearing central chest pain that may radiate into the back. Care is centered around gentle but rapid transport to the trauma center. Oxygen is administered and fluid infusion should be very minimal.

A rupture or penetrating injury to the aorta results in almost immediate death as the vessel is very large and contains great pressure. The patient will have a history of penetrating or severe blunt chest trauma and display the signs of shock and move quickly to decompensation and death. Care is directed to oxygen administration, shock management, and rapid transport to the trauma center.

b. **Vena cava**   **pp. 396–397**

Injury to the vena cava is only slightly less severe than aortic injury since the vessels carry the same volume of fluid, but under different pressures (less for the vena cava). The progression of injury is just slightly slower with injury to the vena cava, though the result of injury is probably the same. In the field, it may be difficult to determine the exact blood vessel involved in a penetrating injury to the chest.

c. **Pulmonary arteries/veins**   **pp. 396–397**

As with aortic and vena caval injuries, the patient will have a history of penetrating or severe blunt trauma and the signs and symptoms of hypovolemia and shock. Care is directed at helping the body compensate for shock, some fluid resuscitation, and rapid transport.

8. **Discuss the pathophysiology of, findings of assessment with, and management and the need for rapid intervention and transport of patients with diaphragmatic, esophageal, and tracheobronchial injuries.**   **pp. 397–398, 410**

Diaphragmatic injury is usually due to severe compression of the diaphragm during blunt abdominal trauma or due to penetrating trauma along the border of the rib cage. Remember that the diaphragm is a dynamic muscle that moves up and down with respiration. Injury may result in less effective respiration and/or the movement of abdominal organs into the chest cavity, most commonly the bowel. The injury may present similarly to tension pneumothorax as the abdominal contents displace the lung tissue. Bowel sounds may also be heard in the chest, though it usually takes too much time to decipher these sounds. Care is directed at treating shock and dyspnea with rapid transport indicated.

Esophageal injury does not usually present with acute symptoms other than a history of penetrating trauma to the central chest. Perforation may permit food, drink, or gastric contents to enter the mediastinum, where it either forms an excellent medium for infection (with gastric contents) or damages some of the structures within. The result is serious damage to some of the most important structures within the chest and a significant mortality rate. The patient with such injury will present with penetrating injury to the region and care is directed toward other, more immediately important pathologies. Nevertheless, suspect esophageal injury and communicate that suspicion to the attending physician.

Tracheobronchial injuries are usually related to penetrating trauma to the upper mediastinum, and they open the major airways to the mediastinum. The injuries permit air to enter the mediastinum and possibly the neck. The patient will have dyspnea (possibly severe) and may have subcutaneous emphysema. Positive-pressure ventilation may make matters worse as air is then actively "pushed" into the mediastinal space. The patient may also experience pneumothorax and tension pneumothorax.

9. **Discuss the pathophysiology of, findings of assessment with, and management and need for rapid intervention and transport of the patient with traumatic asphyxia.**

Traumatic asphyxia is a crushing-type injury in which the crushing mechanism remains in place and restricts both respiration and venous return to the central circulation. The patient may display bulging eyes, petechial hemorrhage, and red or blue skin above the level of compression. The injury may damage many internal blood vessels but tamponades hemorrhage because of the continuing compression. Once the compression is released, profound hypovolemia may occur and the patient may demonstrate the signs and symptoms of serious internal injury. Care is directed at oxygen administration, ventilation, fluid resuscitation, and rapid transport to the trauma center.

10. **Differentiate between thoracic injuries based on the assessment and history.** pp. 398–403

Anterior blunt trauma is most likely to cause rib fracture, pulmonary contusion, closed pneumothorax ("paper bag" syndrome) (possibly progressing to tension pneumothorax), and myocardial contusion. Sharp pain suggests rib fracture, while dull pain suggests pulmonary or myocardial contusion. Dyspnea may be present in all circumstances but will likely be progressive and become severe with pulmonary contusion or pneumothorax. Lateral impact may cause traumatic aortic aneurysm with tearing chest pain, possibly radiating to the back. Crushing injury may cause traumatic asphyxia and display with a discolored upper body and severe shock at the pressure release.

Penetrating trauma may induce an open pneumothorax but is more likely to cause closed pneumothorax unless there is a very large entrance wound. Injury to the great vessels and heart may cause immediate exsanguination, while heart injury may lead to pericardial tamponade. Penetrating trauma to the central chest may perforate any mediastinal structure, including the trachea or esophagus. Rapid hypovolemia and shock suggest great vessel or heart injury, while progressively increasing dyspnea suggests tension pneumothorax. Severe dyspnea, absent breath sounds on the ipsilateral side, and distended jugular veins confirm a probable diagnosis of tension pneumothorax. Any penetration of the thorax with possible entry into the mediastinum should suggest esophageal or tracheal injury.

11. **Given several preprogrammed and moulaged thoracic trauma patients, provide the appropriate scene size-up, initial assessment, focused assessment, detailed assessment and the proper patient care and transport.** pp. 398–410

During your training as an EMT-Paramedic you will participate in many classroom practice sessions involving simulated patients. You will also spend some time in the emergency departments of local hospitals as well as in advanced-level ambulances gaining clinical experience. During these times, use your knowledge of thoracic trauma to help you assess and care for the simulated or real patients you attend.

CASE STUDY REVIEW

Reread the case study on pages 365 and 366 in Paramedic Care: Trauma Emergencies *before reading the discussion below.*

This case study presents many of the important elements of assessment and care for the patient who has suffered penetrating injury to the chest. It identifies the need to recognize and aggressively manage the patient. It also highlights the value of rapid transport, when called for.

The paramedics on Medic 101, Victoria and Christian, use the time during their response to identify their duties, the equipment that will likely by needed, and procedures they may perform. Of primary concern is scene safety for the paramedics, fellow rescuers, bystanders, and the patient, especially since shots have been fired. The paramedics are also concerned about the severity of the injuries that may have resulted. They mentally review the steps of assessment and management of both chest and abdominal injuries. As the rescue unit arrives, it is apparent that the police have secured the scene and concern can be directed to the patient.

The initial assessment of the patient presents only minor signs of injury. The wounds are small and not bleeding severely. The patient does not appear to be in much pain. Victoria and Christian do notice that the patient's level of consciousness and color suggest shock, as do the labored, rapid, and shallow breathing and the patient's ability to speak only in short phrases. Their quick initial assessment reveals reasons to be concerned about the airway (reduced level of consciousness) and breathing (speaking in short phrases and poor color). Circulation is deficient, as the paramedics note the distal pulses are absent and the carotid pulse is rapid and weak. This patient is clearly one who merits a rapid trauma assessment and rapid transport to the trauma center.

The rapid trauma assessment reveals that the patient was struck by four bullets, increasing the likelihood that critical structures were injured. Even though the wounds are small in nature, the paramedics remember the severe injuries a bullet can produce. They also note powder burns and residue on Conrad's shirt due to the proximity of the gun barrel to his chest when it was fired. They carefully remove the shirt without cutting it. (If cutting was required, they would have cut without cutting through the bullet holes.) Their actions help maintain the integrity of the evidence as it may be used in court.

Victoria and Christian quickly cover each wound with an occlusive dressing, sealed on three sides to prevent entry of air into the chest and to permit any air under pressure to escape (as with the development of tension pneumothorax). Their assessment finds full jugular veins, a normal finding in a normovolemic patient in the supine position. The slightly diminished breath sounds on the right side suggest some pneumothorax and reason to perform frequent ongoing assessments evaluating the right side for breath sounds.

Conrad receives care in anticipation of shock including high-flow oxygen and IVs started in each upper extremity with large-bore catheters and macrodrip or trauma tubing. The paramedics also employ spinal precautions with him, just in case one of the bullets has damaged the vertebral column and endangered the spinal cord.

Careful ongoing assessments reveal a continuing degeneration in the patient's condition. This prompts Victoria and Christian to search for a possible cause of the deterioration. Increasingly quieter breath sounds on the right side, hyperinflation of the right side, tracheal deviation (a late and infrequent sign of tension pneumothorax), increasing dyspnea, and overall patient degeneration together suggest a developing pneumothorax, possibly a tension pneumothorax. The team first tries to relieve the condition by unsealing the dressings covering the wound sites. These actions are unsuccessful, so medical direction is contacted and the paramedics receive authorization to perform a needle decompression of the thorax at the second intercostal space, midclavicular line. Victoria places a large-bore (14-gauge) catheter just above the third rib (into the 2nd intercostal space) until she feels a "pop" and hears air rush out. The attempt is successful, as demonstrated by the escaping air. The bullet wound dressings are reapplied and a valve assembly (a cut glove finger) is applied to the needle hub. Then Christian and Victoria watch their patient very carefully during transport for the redevelopment of the tension pneumothorax because they know that the catheter inserted in the chest may kink or clog with blood or other fluid.

CONTENT SELF-EVALUATION

MULTIPLE CHOICE

_____ 1. About what percentage of vehicle deaths are attributable to thoracic injuries?
A. 10
B. 25
C. 35
D. 45
E. 65

_____ 2. Which of the following is located within the thorax?
A. the heart
B. both lungs
C. the esophagus
D. the trachea
E. all of the above

_____ 3. How many rib pairs are floating ribs?
   A. 1
   B. 2
   C. 3
   D. 6
   E. 8

_____ 4. Which of the following lines is used to describe position on the chest wall?
   A. the posterior axillary line
   B. the anterior axillary line
   C. the medial axillary line
   D. the midclavicular line
   E. all of the above

_____ 5. How high does the diaphragm rise in the chest during a maximum inspiration?
   A. to the 2nd intercostal space posteriorly
   B. to the 4th intercostal space posteriorly
   C. to the 6th intercostal space posteriorly
   D. to the 8th intercostal space posteriorly
   E. to the manubrium anteriorly

_____ 6. The muscle(s) of respiration responsible for reducing the distance between ribs and helping lift the thorax is(are) the:
   A. intercostal muscles.
   B. diaphragm.
   C. sternocleidomastoid muscles.
   D. scalene.
   E. rectus abdominis.

_____ 7. The structure that separates the chest cavity from the abdominal cavity is the:
   A. mediastinum.
   B. peritoneum.
   C. perineum.
   D. diaphragm.
   E. vena cava.

_____ 8. At the beginning of and during most of expiration, the pressure within the thorax is:
   A. less than the environment pressure.
   B. more than the environment pressure.
   C. equal to the environment pressure.
   D. first lower than and then higher than the environmental pressure.
   E. first higher than and then lower than the environmental pressure.

_____ 9. Which structures enter or exit the lungs at the pulmonary hilum?
   A. the right mainstem bronchus
   B. the thoracic duct
   C. the pulmonary artery
   D. the pulmonary veins
   E. all except B

_____ 10. The right lung has only two lobes because the heart's greatest mass is on the right.
   A. True
   B. False

_____ 11. The serous structure that ensures the lungs expand with the thoracic cage wall and diaphragm is the:
   A. pleura.
   B. hilum.
   C. ligamentum arteriosum.
   D. lobular attachment.
   E. mediastinum.

_____ 12. The oxygen content of the air we breathe in is:
   A. 79 percent.
   B. 21 percent.
   C. 4 percent.
   D. 0.04 percent.
   E. 16 percent.

_____ 13. The carbon dioxide content of the air we breathe out is:
   A. 79 percent.
   B. 21 percent.
   C. 4 percent.
   D. 0.04 percent.
   E. 16 percent.

_____ 14. The volume of air moved with each normal breath is called the:
    A. residual volume.   D. vital capacity.
    B. dead space volume.   E. inspiratory capacity.
    C. tidal volume.

_____ 15. The maximum volume of air inhaled into the lungs after a normal expiration is called the:
    A. residual volume.   D. vital capacity.
    B. dead space volume.   E. inspiratory capacity.
    C. tidal volume.

_____ 16. Which of the following is used by the central nervous system to regulate respiration?
    A. the level of CO_2 in the cerebrospinal fluid
    B. chemoreceptors in the carotid bodies
    C. chemoreceptors in the medulla oblongata
    D. oxygen levels in the blood
    E. all of the above

_____ 17. Which of the following monitors carbon dioxide levels to institute respiration?
    A. chemoreceptors in the carotid bodies
    B. chemoreceptors in the medulla oblongata
    C. the apneustic center
    D. chemoreceptors in the aortic bodies
    E. both A and D

_____ 18. Which of the following acts as a shut-off switch for respiration?
    A. chemoreceptors in the carotid bodies
    B. chemoreceptors in the medulla oblongata
    C. the apneustic center
    D. chemoreceptors in the aortic bodies
    E. both A and D

_____ 19. Which of the following structures is NOT located within the mediastinum?
    A. the thoracic duct   D. the vagus nerve
    B. the phrenic nerve   E. esophagus
    C. pulmonary hilum

_____ 20. The coronary arteries fill primarily during diastole and are somewhat constricted during systole by the contraction of the myocardium, further limiting blood flow through them.
    A. True
    B. False

_____ 21. Which of the following statements is NOT true regarding the pericardium?
    A. The pericardial fluid is straw colored.
    B. The pericardial fluid acts as a lubricant.
    C. The pericardium normally contains no more than 5 mL of fluid.
    D. The epicardium and visceral pericardium are one and the same.
    E. The fibrous pericardium is not the parietal pericardium.

_____ 22. The smooth interior layer of the heart is the:
    A. fibrous pericardium.   D. endocardium.
    B. epicardium.   E. myocardium.
    C. pericardium.

_____ 23. The outer layer of the heart is the:
    A. fibrous pericardium.   D. endocardium.
    B. epicardium.   E. myocardium.
    C. pericardium.

_____ **24.** The intercostal arteries and nerves run:
  A. behind the ribs.
  B. above the ribs.
  C. in front of the ribs.
  D. under the ribs.
  E. both A and D

_____ **25.** Which of the following is NOT likely to be associated with blunt trauma?
  A. pericardial tamponade
  B. pneumothorax (paper bag syndrome)
  C. traumatic asphyxia
  D. aortic aneurysm
  E. myocardial contusion

_____ **26.** Which of the following is NOT likely to be associated with penetrating trauma?
  A. open pneumothorax
  B. esophageal disruption
  C. traumatic asphyxia
  D. cavitational lung injury
  E. comminuted fracture of the ribs

_____ **27.** Rib fracture is found in about what percent of significant chest trauma?
  A. 10 percent
  B. 25 percent
  C. 35 percent
  D. 50 percent
  E. 65 percent

_____ **28.** Which ribs are fractured the most frequently?
  A. ribs 1 and 3
  B. ribs 4 through 8
  C. ribs 7 through 9
  D. ribs 8 through 11
  E. ribs 9 through 12

_____ **29.** Which rib group results in mortality up to 30 percent when they are fractured?
  A. ribs 1 and 3
  B. ribs 4 through 8
  C. ribs 7 through 9
  D. ribs 8 through 11
  E. ribs 9 through 12

_____ **30.** Which of the following groups is more likely to experience internal injury without rib fracture?
  A. the pediatric patient
  B. the adult male patient
  C. the adult female patient
  D. the elderly female patient
  E. the elderly male patient

_____ **31.** Which of the following is a sign or symptom of rib fracture?
  A. local pain
  B. crepitus
  C. limited chest excursion
  D. hemothorax
  E. all of the above

_____ **32.** Which of the following is most frequently associated with sternal fracture?
  A. hemothorax
  B. myocardial contusion
  C. esophageal injury
  D. simple pneumothorax
  E. open pneumothorax

_____ **33.** Air from under the flail segment in flail chest does which of the following?
  A. moves out from under the segment during expiration
  B. moves toward the segment during expiration
  C. does not move with the segment
  D. moves out from under the segment during inspiration
  E. none of the above

_____ **34.** As the pain of the flail chest increases with time, the amount of paradoxical movement will decrease due to muscular splinting.
  A. True
  B. False

_____ 35. Simple pneumothorax is associated with what percent of serious thoracic trauma?
   A. 5
   B. 10 to 30
   C. 25 to 50
   D. 60
   E. more than 75

_____ 36. The condition in which a part of the chest wall moves in opposition to the rest of the chest due to numerous rib fractures is called:
   A. pneumothorax.
   B. tension pneumothorax.
   C. hemothorax.
   D. atelectasis.
   E. none of the above

_____ 37. The chest injury that causes the patient to experience increasing dyspnea because of an open or closed pneumothorax that has a valve-like function and allows intrathoracic pressure to increase is referred to as:
   A. subcutaneous emphysema.
   B. traumatic asphyxia.
   C. hyperbaric mediastinal displacement.
   D. tension pneumothorax.
   E. flail chest.

_____ 38. For air to move through an open wound to create an open pneumothorax, the wound opening must be:
   A. just large enough to permit air passage.
   B. two-thirds the size of the tracheal opening.
   C. the size of the trachea.
   D. about the size of a hunting rifle bullet.
   E. larger than the trachea.

_____ 39. Which of the following is a very late sign of tension pneumothorax?
   A. head and neck petechiae
   B. intercostal bulging
   C. a narrowing pulse pressure
   D. tracheal deviation away from the injury
   E. distended jugular veins

_____ 40. Each hemithorax can hold up to what volume of blood from a hemothorax?
   A. 500 mL
   B. 750 mL
   C. 1,500 mL
   D. 3,000 mL
   E. 4,500 mL

_____ 41. Which of the following statements is NOT true regarding hemothorax?
   A. Hemorrhage into the thorax is more severe due to decreased pressure there.
   B. Serious hemothorax may displace an entire lung and has a 75 percent mortality rate.
   C. Hemothorax often occurs with pneumothorax.
   D. Hemothorax rarely occurs with simple rib fractures.
   E. none of the above

_____ 42. Distant or absent breath sounds heard during auscultation of the chest and the signs of shock are suggestive of which pathology?
   A. pneumothorax
   B. tension pneumothorax
   C. aortic aneurysm
   D. pulmonary contusion
   E. hemothorax

_____ 43. Which of the following problems would most likely result in a chest area that was dull to percussion?
   A. pneumothorax
   B. tension pneumothorax
   C. hemothorax
   D. subcutaneous pneumothorax
   E. pericardial tamponade

_____ 44. Your patient has received chest trauma yet did not initially present with crackles. However, as the assessment continues, they are heard in both the lower lung fields. This condition is most likely a result of which of the following?
A. pulmonary contusion
B. hemothorax
C. pneumothorax
D. aortic aneurysm
E. pericardial tamponade

_____ 45. Extensive pulmonary contusions may account for blood losses up to 1,500 mL.
A. True
B. False

_____ 46. The most common cause of myocardial contusion is:
A. blunt anterior chest trauma.
B. blunt lateral chest trauma.
C. penetrating anterior chest trauma.
D. blunt posterior chest trauma.
E. the pressure wave of an explosion.

_____ 47. A patient presents with the signs of shock, jugular vein distention, distant heart sounds, and a narrowing pulse pressure. The lung fields are clear. Which condition is most likely the cause?
A. tension pneumothorax
B. hemothorax
C. traumatic asphyxia
D. pericardial tamponade
E. atelectasis

_____ 48. Pericardial tamponade occurs with what frequency in serious chest trauma patients?
A. less than 2 percent of the time
B. 10 percent of the time
C. 20 percent of the time
D. 25 percent of the time
E. 30 to 45 percent of the time

_____ 49. Which of the following is a sign of pericardial tamponade?
A. pulsus paradoxus
B. a narrowing pulse pressure
C. distended jugular veins
D. hypotension
E. all of the above

_____ 50. The patient with pericardial tamponade may be in hypovolemic shock due to the volume of blood lost into the pericardial sac.
A. True
B. False

_____ 51. A decrease in jugular vein distention during inspiration is known as:
A. Beck's triad.
B. pulsus paradoxus.
C. Cushing's reflex.
D. Kussmaul's sign.
E. electrical alternans.

_____ 52. A blood pressure drop of more than 10 mmHg with inspiration is known as:
A. Beck's triad.
B. pulsus paradoxus.
C. Cushing's reflex.
D. Kussmaul's sign.
E. electrical alternans.

_____ 53. If the chamber of the heart is significantly damaged yet does not rupture immediately, it is likely to rupture in around two weeks.
A. True
B. False

_____ 54. Your patient was involved in a lateral impact auto accident. The car is greatly deformed, though the patient does not have many signs of injury. During your assessment, he complains of a tearing sensation in his central chest and numbness in his left upper extremity. Your highest index of suspicion of injury is for:
A. traumatic asphyxia.
B. pulmonary contusion.
C. aortic aneurysm.
D. myocardial contusion.
E. pericardial tamponade.

_____ 55. What percentage of patients with traumatic aortic aneurysm survive the initial impact and injury?
A. as high as 10 percent
B. as high as 20 percent
C. 50 percent
D. 70 percent
E. 73 percent

_____ 56. In a patient with a history of blunt lateral trauma and a suspected traumatic aortic aneurysm, which signs or symptoms would you expect to find?
A. severe tearing chest pain
B. pulse deficit between extremities
C. reduced pulse strength in the lower extremities
D. hypertension
E. all of the above

_____ 57. A harsh systolic murmur is heard over the central chest. This is suggestive of which pathology?
A. pneumothorax
B. tension pneumothorax
C. traumatic aortic aneurysm
D. pulmonary contusion
E. hemothorax

_____ 58. The right side is the site of most diaphragmatic ruptures as most assailants are right-handed.
A. True
B. False

_____ 59. The traumatic diaphragmatic rupture is likely to present like which of the following thoracic injuries?
A. tension pneumothorax
B. pulmonary contusion
C. aortic aneurysm
D. pericardial tamponade
E. esophageal injury

_____ 60. The two major problems associated with traumatic asphyxia are restriction of chest excursion and:
A. distortion of the airway.
B. restriction of venous return.
C. atelectasis.
D. hemorrhage during the compression.
E. massive strokes.

_____ 61. The classic signs of traumatic asphyxia include which of the following?
A. bulging eyes
B. conjunctival hemorrhage
C. petechiae of the head and neck
D. dark red or purple appearance of the head and neck
E. all of the above

_____ 62. Serious penetrating trauma will likely require which of the following body substance isolation procedures?
A. gloves
B. face shield
C. gown
D. mask
E. all of the above

_____ 63. During your assessment of a supine patient with blunt chest trauma, you notice slight jugular vein distention. With no other signs of injury, this suggests which of the following?
A. a normal patient
B. pericardial tamponade
C. tension pneumothorax
D. traumatic asphyxia
E. B, C, and D

_____ 64. Crackles heard during auscultation of the chest are suggestive of which pathology?
A. pneumothorax
B. tension pneumothorax
C. aortic aneurysm
D. pulmonary contusion
E. hemothorax

_____ 65. Hyperresonance heard during percussion of the chest is suggestive of which pathology?
A. pneumothorax
B. tension pneumothorax
C. hemothorax
D. pulmonary contusion
E. both A and B

_____ 66. Which of the following thoracic structures takes the least energy to fracture and often results as a more common, yet less serious, thoracic injury?
A. ribs 1 through 3
B. ribs 4 through 9
C. ribs 10 through 12
D. the sternum
E. the manubrium

_____ 67. A patient who displays subcutaneous emphysema is most likely to have which of the conditions listed below?
A. traumatic asphyxia
B. tension pneumothorax
C. the paper bag syndrome
D. pulmonary contusion
E. cardiac contusion

_____ 68. Overdrive ventilation (bag-valve masking) of the patient with flail chest will cause the flail segment to move with, rather than in opposition to, the chest wall.
A. True
B. False

_____ 69. Which of the following is an indication for the use of PASG?
A. diaphragmatic rupture
B. penetrating chest injury
C. blunt chest trauma with a blood pressure below 100
D. blunt chest trauma with a blood pressure below 60
E. suspected pericardial tamponade

_____ 70. Meperidine, diazepam, or morphine may be given the minor rib fracture patient to reduce pain and increase respiratory excursion.
A. True
B. False

_____ 71. The patient who is suspected of a flail chest or other thoracic cage injury, without suspected spine injury, should be positioned:
A. on the uninjured side.
B. on the injured side.
C. supine with legs elevated.
D. on the left lateral side.
E. on the right lateral side.

_____ 72. The open pneumothorax should be cared for using which of the following techniques?
A. Pack the wound with a sterile dressing.
B. Cover the wound an occlusive dressing and tape securely.
C. Cover the wound with an occlusive dressing, taped on three sides.
D. Attempt to close the wound with a hemostat and then cover with a sterile dressing.
E. Cover the wound loosely with a sterile dressing.

_____ 73. Which location is recommended for prehospital pleural decompression?
A. 2nd intercostal space, midclavicular line
B. 5th intercostal space, midclavicular line
C. 5th intercostal space, midaxillary line
D. A and B
E. A and C

_____ 74. A few minutes after you have inserted a needle and decompressed a tension pneumothorax, you notice that a patient's dyspnea is getting worse and breath sounds on the injured side are becoming diminished. Which action would you take?
A. Insert a second needle.
B. Remove the dressing.
C. Provide overdrive ventilation.
D. Consider nitrous oxide administration.
E. all of the above

_____ **75.** A patient is trapped in a wrecked auto for about half an hour and is suspected of having traumatic asphyxia. Care should include which of the following?
   A. two large-bore IVs
   B. normal saline or lactated Ringer's solution
   C. fluids run rapidly
   D. consideration of sodium bicarbonate
   E. all of the above

SPECIAL PROJECTS

Labeling Diagrams

I. Write the names of the organs and structures of the thorax marked A, B, C, D, E, F, G, and H in the figure below.

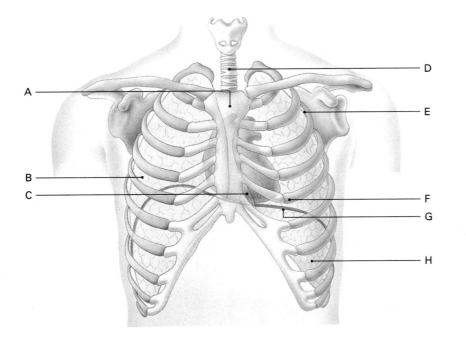

A. _____

B. _____

C. _____

D. _____

E. _____

F. _____

G. _____

H. _____

II. Match the labels A through K on the accompanying diagram to the following respiration volumes.

_____ **1.** Inspiratory reserve   _____ **7.** Inspiratory capacity

_____ **2.** Expiratory reserve   _____ **8.** Functional reserve capacity

_____ **3.** Residual volume   _____ **9.** Normal respiration

_____ **4.** Vital capacity   _____ **10.** Maximum inspiration

_____ **5.** Tidal volume   _____ **11.** Maximum expiration

_____ **6.** Total lung capacity

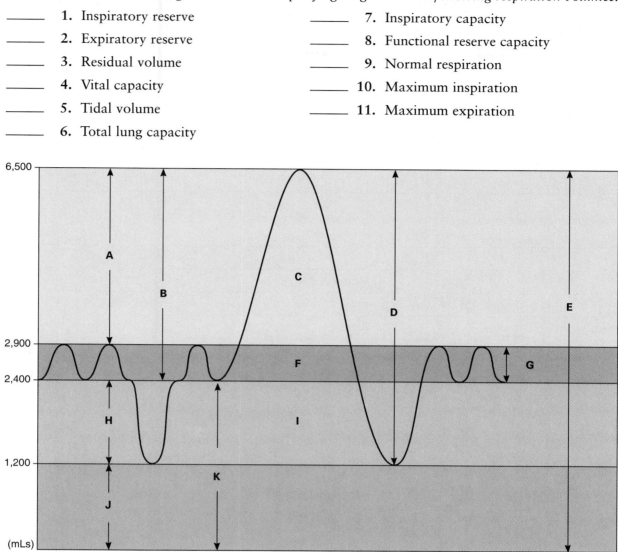

Problem Solving—Chest Injury

One of the more serious respiratory-related emergencies is the tension pneumothorax. Identify the signs and symptoms you would expect to find in a patient with this pathology and its increasing intrathoracic pressure.

_____

_____

_____

_____

_____

_____

_____

Give a patient report to medical direction based upon the signs and symptoms identified above. Use only that information you feel important for the medical direction physician. (You are attempting to receive permission to provide pleural decompression.)

_____

_____

_____

_____

_____

_____

Identify the exact location of your decompression attempt.

_____

_____

_____

_____

CHAPTER 11
*
Abdominal Trauma

Review of Chapter Objectives

After reading this chapter, you should be able to:

1. **Describe the epidemiology, including the morbidity/mortality, for patients with abdominal trauma as well as prevention strategies to avoid the injuries.**   **pp. 414–415**

   While serious abdominal trauma accounts for some mortality, it ranks behind head and chest trauma as a region associated with trauma deaths. Rapid transport to the trauma center and modern surgical techniques have accounted for a great decrease in abdominal trauma mortality and morbidity, but it still remains a serious consideration during trauma assessment and care. Highway and vehicle design and the proper use of restraints have reduced abdominal injuries greatly, however, and more correct use of seat belts by greater numbers of the population can lead to continuing decreases in both the incidence and severity of abdominal injury.

2. **Apply epidemiologic principles to develop prevention strategies for abdominal injuries.**   **p. 415**

   The current major causes of abdominal injury are improper seat belt use and violence. Education programs designed to promote the use and proper application of seat belts and programs to reduce unintentional or deliberate injuries resulting from handguns can help further reduce abdominal injury.

3. **Describe the anatomy and physiology of organs and structures related to abdominal injuries.**   **pp. 415–425**

   The abdomen is one of the body's largest cavities, bounded superiorly by the diaphragm, laterally by the flank muscles, inferiorly by the pelvis, posteriorly by the spine and back muscles, and anteriorly by the abdominal muscles. Since most of its border is soft tissue, it is rather unprotected from injury. The abdomen contains the continuous, muscular tube of digestion, the alimentary canal. It enters the abdomen through the hiatus of the diaphragm as the esophagus. It joins the stomach, an organ that physically mixes the food with gastric juices and then sends it out and into the small bowel. The first portion of the bowel, the duodenum, mixes the digesting food with bile (a byproduct of the liver) and pancreatic juices and then begins the process of absorption. The remainder of the small bowel draws the nutrients from the food.

   As the digesting food enters the large bowel it is mixed with bacteria, releasing water and any remaining nutrients. They are absorbed, and the material is pushed by peristalsis to the rectum, awaiting defecation. The bowel is a thin and vascular tube that drains its blood supply through the liver for detoxification, where some nutrients are stored and others added to the circulation.

   The liver is a large, solid organ found in the right upper quadrant, just below the diaphragm. The pancreas is a delicate organ found in the lower aspect of the upper left quadrant with a portion of it extending into the right upper quadrant. In addition to digestive juices, it manufactures insulin and glucagon. The kidneys are found deep within the flanks and filter blood to remove excess water and electrolytes. They are very vascular organs that excrete urine into the ureters through which the urine then travels to the bladder. The bladder (in the central pelvic space) rids the body of urine through the urethra. The spleen is an organ of the immune system and is very delicate and vascular, residing in the left upper quadrant.

The abdominal cavity is lined with a serous membrane, the peritoneum. It covers the anterior abdominal organs and a double-layer sheath of it forms the omentum, which covers the anterior surface of the abdomen. The bowel is slung from the posterior wall of the abdomen by connective tissue called the mesentery that also provides perfusion to the bowel. The abdominal aorta and inferior vena cava run along the spinal column and branch frequently to serve the abdominal organs.

4. Predict abdominal injuries based on blunt and penetrating mechanisms of injury. pp. 425–433

Blunt trauma compresses, shears, or decelerates the various organs and structures within the abdomen resulting in rupture of the hollow organs, fracture or tearing of the solid organs, or tearing or severance of the abdominal vasculature. The spleen is the most frequently injured organ with the liver the second most commonly injured structure. The bowel, kidneys, and diaphragm are also common recipients of blunt injury.

Penetrating injury to the abdomen may involve low- and high-velocity objects. Bullets disrupt a larger cylinder of tissue with their passage and are especially damaging to hollow organs filled with fluid and to the extremely dense and delicate solid organs of the abdomen. Mortality is about ten times greater with high-energy bullets than with stab-type wounds. The liver is affected more frequently than the bowel, with the spleen, kidneys, and pancreas injured in descending order of frequency. A special category of penetrating injury is the shotgun blast. At short range (under 3 yards), the projectiles have tremendous energy and create numerous tracts of serious injury.

5. Describe open and closed abdominal injuries. pp. 425–428

Open wounds to the abdomen may be very small, such as those caused by a bullet or knife, or large enough to permit abdominal contents to protrude (an evisceration). Bullet wounds may cause injury beyond their direct path through cavitation and are especially harmful to the solid organs (liver, spleen, kidneys, pancreas) or to the stomach and intestinal tract when full of fluid. Shotgun blasts, especially if delivered from less than 7 feet, are extremely damaging because the many small projectiles still have significant kinetic energy and have not yet spread out to disperse their energy.

Blunt (closed) injuries may compress the internal organs of the abdomen between the offending object and the spine or posterior abdominal wall or between other organs. The force may shear solid organs and their vascular attachments or may directly cause organ fracture and hemorrhage or the spillage of organ contents or both. Hollow organs may rupture and spill their contents into the abdominal cavity. Severe abdominal compression may rupture the diaphragm and push abdominal organs into the thorax.

6. Identify the need for rapid intervention and transport of the patient with abdominal injuries based on assessment findings. pp. 433–439

The abdomen, for the most part, is bound by connective and muscle tissue rather than the skeletal structures found protecting the skull and thorax. This permits an easier transmission of traumatic forces to the internal organs and frequent injury. The abdomen also does not show the dramatic signs and symptoms of injury seen elsewhere, again because of the lack of rigid skeletal protection. Hence, it is important to carefully assess the abdominal cavity, looking for any sign of trauma (such as erythema), and to question the patient about pain or other abdominal symptoms. Blood, bacteria, and, to a lesser degree, gastric, duodenal, and pancreatic contents irritate the abdominal lining (the peritoneum) only after the passage of time, which again limits the signs and symptoms of serious abdominal injury visible during prehospital care.

7. **Explain the pathophysiology of solid and hollow organ injuries, abdominal vascular injuries, pelvic fractures, and other abdominal injuries.** pp. 428–433

Solid Organ Injuries

The spleen is well protected, although it is very delicate and not contained within a strong capsule. It frequently ruptures and bleeds heavily. The liver is a very dense and vascular organ in the right upper quadrant just behind the lower border of the rib cage. It is contained within a strong capsule, although it can be lacerated during severe deceleration by its restraining ligament (the ligamentum teres). The kidneys are well protected both by their location deep within the flank and by strong capsules. The pancreas is located in the lower portion of the left upper quadrant, extending just into the right quadrant. It is more delicate than either the liver or kidneys even though it lies deep within the central abdomen. When injured, it may hemorrhage and release pancreatic juices into the abdomen.

Hollow Organ Injuries

Hollow organs include the stomach, small and large bowel, rectum, gall bladder, urinary bladder, and pregnant uterus. Compression may contuse them or cause them to rupture while penetrating injury may perforate them. The gall bladder, stomach, and first part of the small bowel may release digestive juices that will chemically irritate and damage the abdominal structures. Injury can cause the rest of the bowel to release material high in bacterial load that can induce infection. The rupture of the urinary bladder will release blood and urine into the abdomen. Injury to the abdomen may cause blood in emesis (hematemesis), blood in the stool (hematochezia), or blood in the urine (hematuria).

Abdominal Vascular Injuries

The major vascular structures of the abdomen include the abdominal aorta, the inferior vena cava, and many arteries branching to the abdominal organs. These vessels may be injured by blunt trauma, though penetrating trauma is a far more frequent cause of injury. The abdomen does not develop an internal pressure against hemorrhage as do the muscles and other solid regions of the body, and bleeding may continue unabated while the accumulation of blood is difficult to recognize.

Pelvic Fractures

Pelvic fractures are addressed in Chapter 7, "Musculoskeletal Trauma," of this volume. However, remember that pelvic fracture can cause injury to the bladder, genitalia, and rectum, and to some very large blood vessels with serious associated hemorrhage.

Other Abdominal Organ Injuries

Other injuries include injuries to the mesentery and peritoneum. The mesentery supports the bowel and may be injured, most commonly at points of fixation like the ileocecal or duodenal/jejunal junctures. Hemorrhage here is often contained by the peritoneum. Peritoneal injury is generally related to irritation either by chemical action (most rapid) or by bacterial contamination (12 to 24 hours).

8. **Describe the assessment findings associated with and management of solid and hollow organ injuries, abdominal vascular injuries, pelvic fractures, and other abdominal injuries.** pp. 433–442

Injury to the abdominal contents is difficult to ascertain because the signs and symptoms of injury are often diffuse and around 30 percent of patients with serious abdominal injury have no clear signs or symptoms of injury. During assessment, you should seek to discover what evidence of injury exists and what it suggests about the injury's precise nature and location. Pay attention to pain, tenderness, and rebound tenderness in each quadrant and note any thirst or other signs of hypovolemia and shock.

The management of the patient with suspected abdominal trauma is basically supportive with airway maintenance, oxygen, ventilation as needed, and fluid resuscitation. Establish large-bore IVs but do not run fluids aggressively unless the blood pressure drops below 100 mmHg. Use of the PASG may be helpful, especially if the blood pressure drops below 50 mmHg. Cover any evisceration with a sterile dressing soaked in normal saline and cover that with an occlusive dressing to prevent evaporation. As with all hypovolemia patients, keep the patient warm and provide rapid transport.

9. **Differentiate between abdominal injuries based on the assessment and history. pp. 427–439**

As mentioned earlier, 30 percent of patients with serious abdominal injury present without signs and symptoms. Many others present with diffuse signs and symptoms, making it very hard to differentiate among the different abdominal pathologies. Try to relate the mechanism of injury or any patient complaints to the anatomic region involved and the specific organs found there. For example, left flank trauma and pain may suggest splenic injury, while right upper quadrant injury and pain may suggest liver pathology.

Penetrating abdominal trauma will present with an entrance wound and, possibly, an exit wound. It may also manifest with the signs and symptoms of blunt abdominal trauma due to the same mechanisms. Evisceration will be evident by the protrusion of bowel from an open wound involving the abdominal wall.

Blunt abdominal trauma may be recognized by abdominal tenderness, rebound tenderness, pain, or a pulsing mass. It may involve any of the abdominal or retroperitoneal organs. Signs will be superficial such as contusions or, more likely, erythema. Symptoms may result from the injury or from blood, body fluids, or bacteria (causing delayed pain) in the peritoneal cavity.

10. **Given several preprogrammed and moulaged patients with simulated abdominal injuries, provide the appropriate assessment, care, and transport.   pp. 433–442**

During your training as an EMT-Paramedic you will participate in many classroom practice sessions involving simulated patients. You will also spend some time in the emergency departments of local hospitals as well as in advanced-level ambulances gaining clinical experience. During these times, use your knowledge of abdominal trauma to help you assess and care for the simulated or real patients you attend.

CASE STUDY REVIEW

Reread the case study on pages 413 and 414 in Paramedic Care: Trauma Emergencies *before reading the discussion below.*

This case study permits us to examine the relevant components of the assessment and care of a patient who has sustained a penetrating injury to the abdomen.

Doug and Janice respond to a domestic disturbance with "shots fired." They appreciate the danger associated with this scene and approach with caution. Only after they are told by police that the scene is safe do they enter and begin their assessment and care. They don gloves and prepare to attend penetrating wounds. When they perform their initial assessment, they note that Marty is conscious, alert, and fully oriented. He is speaking in full sentences and appears in no serious or immediate distress. From this, they determine that he has a patent airway and breathing is adequate. They quickly check his pulse and find it strong and regular at 80. Janice quickly visualizes the wound and determines that there is no serious external hemorrhage, though she appreciates the likelihood of serious continuing internal blood loss. Marty quickly looks for an expected exit wound in the flanks or back but finds none. They apply oxygen via nonrebreather mask and apply a pulse oximeter that immediately reveals a saturation of 99 percent. They plan for rapid transport to the hospital (a trauma center) as they begin their focused assessment.

Marty's description of his pain is classic for an abdominal injury. The expanding "burning" pain and the tenderness are suggestive of peritonitis caused as bowel or gastric contents spread into the peritoneal space. Janice covers the small wound with a dressing and prepares Marty for rapid transport. En route, Janice auscultates the abdomen (though she knows she is unlikely to hear bowel sounds) and does likewise to the lower chest as she wishes to rule out chest penetration. Remember that the diaphragm moves up and down in the region of the thoracic border and that bullets frequently deflect from a straight path.

Once the rapid trauma assessment is complete, Janice initiates an IV line with a large catheter and trauma tubing and runs lactated Ringer's solution at a moderate rate. If Marty begins to show signs of hypovolemia and vascular compensation, she will open the flow wide and may consider the inflation of the PASG. Ongoing assessments begin to suggest shock compensation, with the pulse rate rising from 80 to 86 to 88 (though it remains strong). The systolic blood pressure remains at 112, but the diastolic is rising from 86 to 92 (a decreasing pulse pressure), suggesting increasing peripheral vasoconstriction and shock compensation. Marty's shallow respirations also suggest continuing blood loss and developing shock. As this team arrives at the emergency department, it will be very important for them to report these findings and describe both the shooting scene (including the weapon caliber) and wound appearance to the attending physician.

CONTENT SELF-EVALUATION

MULTIPLE CHOICE

_____ 1. Which of the following abdominal organs is found in the left upper quadrant?
A. the spleen
B. the gallbladder
C. the appendix
D. sigmoid colon
E. the liver

_____ 2. Which of the following abdominal organs is found in the right lower quadrant?
A. the spleen
B. the gallbladder
C. the appendix
D. sigmoid colon
E. the liver

_____ 3. Which of the following abdominal organs is found in all of the abdominal quadrants?
A. the pancreas
B. the gallbladder
C. the appendix
D. sigmoid colon
E. small bowel

_____ 4. Which of the following statements is TRUE regarding the digestive tract?
A. It is 25-foot-long hollow tube.
B. It churns food.
C. It introduces digestive juices.
D. It moves food via peristalsis.
E. all of the above

_____ 5. In what order does digesting food pass through the digestive tract?
A. duodenum, ileum, jejunum, colon
B. duodenum, jejunum, ileum, colon
C. jejunum, ileum, colon, duodenum
D. ileum, jejunum, colon, duodenum
E. colon, jejunum, ileum, duodenum

_____ 6. The movement of digesting material through the digestive system occurs through a process called:
A. peristalsis.
B. chyme.
C. peritonitis.
D. emulsification.
E. evisceration.

_____ 7. The largest solid organ of the abdomen is the:
A. spleen.
B. small bowel.
C. pancreas.
D. gallbladder.
E. liver.

_____ 8. The delicate vascular organ that performs some immune functions is the:
A. spleen.
B. small bowel.
C. pancreas.
D. gallbladder.
E. liver.

_____ 9. The solid organ that produces insulin, glucagon, and some digestive juices is the:
A. spleen.
B. small bowel.
C. pancreas.
D. gallbladder.
E. liver.

_____ 10. The urinary bladder may contain as little as 100 mL of fluid or as much as 2,000 mL of fluid.
   A. True
   B. False

_____ 11. The genital structure that contains the developing fetus during gestation is the:
   A. vagina.   D. ovary.
   B. uterus.   E. cervix.
   C. fallopian tube.

_____ 12. The genital structure that releases an egg every 28 days is the:
   A. vagina.   D. ovary.
   B. uterus.   E. cervix.
   C. fallopian tube.

_____ 13. At what point does the uterus and developing fetus fill the abdominal cavity to the lower rib margin?
   A. 12 weeks   D. 40 weeks
   B. 20 weeks   E. 52 weeks
   C. 32 weeks

_____ 14. Pregnancy causes what change in the maternal blood volume?
   A. a 10 percent decrease   D. a 45 percent increase
   B. a 25 percent decrease   E. a 65 percent increase
   C. a 25 percent increase

_____ 15. The abdominal aorta divides into what arteries as it enters the pelvic cavity?
   A. the femoral arteries   D. the phrenic arteries
   B. the innominate arteries   E. the renal arteries
   C. the iliac arteries

_____ 16. The serous lining of the abdominal cavity is the:
   A. perineum.   D. retroperitoneum.
   B. mesentery.   E. ileum.
   C. peritoneum.

_____ 17. Which of the following is a retroperitoneal organ?
   A. the small bowel   D. kidneys
   B. the liver   E. sigmoid colon
   C. the urinary bladder

_____ 18. Due to the anatomy of the abdomen, injury to its contents often presents with limited signs and symptoms.
   A. True
   B. False

_____ 19. Bullets cause an abdominal wound mortality rate that is about equal to that caused by slow-moving penetrating objects.
   A. True
   B. False

_____ 20. Penetrating mechanisms of injury are responsible for what percentage of injuries to the liver?
   A. 50 percent   D. 20 percent
   B. 40 percent   E. 10 percent
   C. 30 percent

_____ 21. Blunt mechanisms of injury are responsible for what percentage of injuries to the liver?
   A. 50 percent   D. 20 percent
   B. 40 percent   E. 10 percent
   C. 30 percent

_____ 22. Which of the following organs is most frequently damaged during blunt abdominal trauma?
  A. the small bowel   D. the kidneys
  B. the liver   E. the pancreas
  C. the spleen

_____ 23. The abdomen is the area for greatest concern when the patient is exposed to severe blast forces.
  A. True
  B. False

_____ 24. Penetration of the abdominal wall resulting in protrusion of the abdominal contents is called:
  A. peristalsis.   D. emulsification.
  B. chyme.   E. evisceration.
  C. peritonitis.

_____ 25. The abdominal organs, with deep expiration, move as far up into the thorax as:
  A. the xiphoid process.   D. the seventh intercostal space.
  B. the tips of the floating ribs. E. none of the above
  C. the nipple line.

_____ 26. The term describing frank blood in the stool is:
  A. hematochezia.   D. hematuria.
  B. hematemesis.   E. hematocrit.
  C. hemoptysis.

_____ 27. The organ most likely to be injured by left flank blunt trauma is:
  A. the small bowel.   D. the kidneys.
  B. the liver.   E. the pancreas.
  C. the spleen.

_____ 28. The organ that is likely to be injured in severe deceleration as its ligament restrains, then lacerates it is:
  A. the small bowel.   D. the kidneys.
  B. the liver.   E. the pancreas.
  C. the spleen.

_____ 29. Most abdominal vascular injuries are associated with penetrating trauma.
  A. True
  B. False

_____ 30. Hemorrhage into the abdomen is of serious concern because it:
  A. quickly puts pressure on internal organs.
  B. limits respirations.
  C. rapidly affects the heart.
  D. may trigger a vagal response, slowing the heart.
  E. none of the above

_____ 31. Blunt injury to the mesentery often occurs at:
  A. the gastric-duodenal juncture.   D. the ileocecal juncture.
  B. the duodenal-jejunal juncture.   E. both B and C
  C. the jejunal-ileal juncture.

_____ 32. How long does it take bacteria to grow in sufficient numbers to irritate the peritoneum?
  A. 2 to 4 hours   D. 8 to 10 hours
  B. 4 to 6 hours   E. over 12 hours
  C. 6 to 8 hours

_____ 33. The number one killer of pregnant females is:
  A. heart attack.   D. trauma.
  B. ectopic pregnancy.   E. stroke.
  C. allergic reactions.

_____ 34. Unrestrained pregnant occupants in vehicles are how many more times likely to suffer fetal mortality in an auto collision than their belted counterparts?
A. two
B. three
C. four
D. five
E. six

_____ 35. The late-term pregnant female is at increased risk for vomiting and aspiration.
A. True
B. False

_____ 36. Supine positioning of the mother may cause hypotension due to:
A. compression of the inferior vena cava.
B. increased circulation to the uterus.
C. increased intra-abdominal pressure.
D. decreased intra-abdominal pressure.
E. Kussmaul's respirations.

_____ 37. It may take a maternal blood loss of what percentage before the heart rate begins to increase in the late term pregnancy?
A. 10 to 15 percent
B. 15 to 20 percent
C. 20 to 25 percent
D. 25 to 30 percent
E. 30 to 35 percent

_____ 38. Due to the flexibility of the pediatric thorax, which injury is more likely to occur with blunt trauma?
A. liver injury
B. splenic injury
C. kidney injury
D. all of the above
E. none of the above

_____ 39. Children may not show signs of blood loss until they have lost what percentage of their volume?
A. 25 percent
B. 35 percent
C. 45 percent
D. 50 percent
E. 65 percent

_____ 40. What percentage of patients with abdominal injury do not present with any signs or symptoms?
A. 10 percent
B. 20 percent
C. 30 percent
D. 40 percent
E. 50 percent

_____ 41. Blunt injury to the right flank region is likely to cause which of the following?
A. liver injury
B. kidney injury
C. bowel injury
D. bladder injury
E. colon injury

_____ 42. Penetrating injury to the central anterior abdomen is likely to cause which of the following?
A. liver injury
B. spleen injury
C. bowel injury
D. bladder injury
E. none of the above

_____ 43. Hemorrhage into the abdomen may account for how much blood loss before it becomes noticeable?
A. 500 mL
B. 750 mL
C. 1,000 mL
D. 1,500 mL
E. 2,500 mL

_____ 44. Prehospital administration of IV fluid should be limited to:
A. 1,000 mL.
B. 2,000 mL.
C. 3,000 mL.
D. 4,000 mL.
E. 5,000 mL.

_____ **45.** Care for the abdominal evisceration includes use of which of the following?
  A. a dry adherent dressing
  B. a dry nonadherent dressing
  C. a sterile dressing moistened with normal saline
  D. an occlusive dressing
  E. a sterile cotton gauze dressing

_____ **46.** At what blood pressure would you consider applying the PASG in the presence of an abdominal evisceration?
  A. 120 mmHg   **D.** 50 mmHg
  B. 100 mmHg   **E.** 30 mmHg
  C. 90 mmHg

_____ **47.** Which position is indicated for the late pregnancy patient?
  A. supine   **D.** Trendelenburg
  B. left lateral recumbent   **E.** with the head elevated 30 degrees
  C. right lateral recumbent

_____ **48.** Use of the PASG is contraindicated in:
  A. geriatric patients.   **D.** abdominal evisceration patients.
  B. patients with low blood pressure.   **E.** diabetic patients.
  C. tuberculosis patients.

_____ **49.** Aggressive fluid resuscitation may aggravate the relative anemia associated with late term pregnancy.
  A. True
  B. False

_____ **50.** Use of the PASG may be beneficial for the patient in early (first-term) pregnancy.
  A. True
  B. False

SPECIAL PROJECT

Writing a Run Report

Writing the run report is one the most important tasks you will perform as a paramedic. Reread the case study on pages 413 and 414 of Paramedic Care: Trauma Emergencies, _and then read the additional information about the call provided below. From this information complete the run report for this call._

The 911 Center dispatches Unit 95 to the Harborview Apartments, Apartment #112 at 3:25 AM. Janice and Doug arrive on scene at 3:32 and finish their first set of vitals at 3:35 as oxygen is applied. Marty is moved to the stretcher a minute later and then to the ambulance. The team departs the scene at 3:38 and is diverted to St. Joseph's Hospital. Janice starts an IV en route with a 14-gauge angiocatheter in the right antecubital fossa, running at about 200 mL/hr. A second set of vitals is taken at 3:42 and finds Marty still fully oriented. Janice questions Marty to find he has a history of seizures but is taking his Dilantin and phenobarbital. He has no allergies and his most recent tetanus shot was 3 years ago. Janice finishes her last set of vitals as they back into St. Joseph's Emergency Department at 3:47. The team fills out its report and radios back in service at 4:00.

Date	Emergency Medical Services Run Report	Run # 914

Patient Information	Service Information	Times

Name:	Agency:	Rcvd	:
Address:	Location:	Enrt	:
City: St: Zip:	Call Origin:	Scne	:
Age: Birth: / / Sex: [M][F]	Type: Emrg [ ] Non [ ] Trnsfr [ ]	LvSn	:
Nature of Call:		ArHsp	:
Chief Complaint:		InSv	:

Description of Current Problem:

Medical Problems

Past		Present
[ ]	Cardiac	[ ]
[ ]	Stroke	[ ]
[ ]	Acute Abdomen	[ ]
[ ]	Diabetes	[ ]
[ ]	Psychiatric	[ ]
[ ]	Epilepsy	[ ]
[ ]	Drug/Alcohol	[ ]
[ ]	Poisoning	[ ]
[ ]	Allergy/Asthma	[ ]
[ ]	Syncope	[ ]
[ ]	Obstetrical	[ ]
[ ]	GYN	[ ]

Other:

Trauma Scr: Glasgow:

On Scene Care:	First Aid:
	By Whom?

02 @ L : Via	C-Collar :	S-Immob. :	Stretcher :

Allergies/Meds:	Past Med Hx:

Time	Pulse	Resp.	BP S/D	LOC	ECG
:	R: [r][i]	R: [s][l]	/	[a][v][p][u]	
Care/Comments:					
:	R: [r][i]	R: [s][l]	/	[a][v][p][u]	
Care/Comments:					
:	R: [r][i]	R: [s][l]	/	[a][v][p][u]	
Care/Comments:					
:	R: [r][i]	R: [s][l]	/	[a][v][p][u]	
Care/Comments:					

Destination:	Personnel:	Certification
Reason: [ ] pt [ ] Closest [ ] M.D. [ ] Other	1.	[P][E][O]
Contacted: [ ] Radio [ ] Tele [ ] Direct	2.	[P][E][O]
Ar Status: [ ] Better [ ] UnC [ ] Worse	3.	[P][E][O]

CHAPTER 12

Shock Trauma Resuscitation

Review of Chapter Objectives

After reading this chapter, you should be able to:

1. Identify the morbidity and mortality associated with blunt and penetrating trauma. **pp. 446–447**

Trauma accounts for about 150,000 deaths yearly, with auto crashes killing around 44,000 and penetrating trauma responsible for another 38,000. While trauma is the number four killer behind heart disease, stroke, and cancer, it is the number one cause of death for individuals under 44 years of age and may be the most expensive heath care problem in our nation today. A particular problem associated with trauma death is the high incidence among young adult males between 13 and 35 years of age. They account for a disproportionate number of trauma deaths (over 30%). This age group needs the special attention of EMS educational efforts.

2. Explain the concept, value, and elements of injury prevention programs. **pp. 447–449**

EMS has not yet embraced the concept of prevention as has the fire service, though prevention shows the greatest promise for reducing the death toll from many types of trauma. More programs promoting responsible and defensive driving, seat belt and helmet use, home safety, and home and workplace safe practices show great potential for reducing the mortality and morbidity from many of the major causes of trauma death. Some progressive emergency service systems have begun programs that go out to the public and make people aware of the steps they can take to make their homes more safe, to drive in safer way, and the make their workplaces more safe. Other agencies and groups are already providing focused programs like "don't drink and drive," "let's not meet by accident," or similar programs.

3. Describe assessment of seriously and nonseriously injured trauma patients. **pp. 449–468**

The assessment of the trauma patient follows the standard prehospital assessment: the scene size-up, the initial assessment, the rapid trauma assessment or focused exam and history, the detailed physical exam (as needed), and then serial ongoing assessments. The seriously injured patient will receive the rapid trauma assessment and quick transport to the trauma center, while the nonseriously injured patient will receive the focused exam and history. The detailed physical exam is reserved for the unusual circumstance where you are searching for the signs and symptoms of other injuries, as in an unconscious patient with care offered for known injuries and a mechanism of injury that would suggest multiple injuries.

4. Identify the aspects of assessment performed during the scene size-up, initial assessment, rapid trauma assessment, focused assessment and history, detailed physical exam, and ongoing assessment for the trauma patient. **pp. 451–468**

The assessment of the trauma patient follows the standard format for assessment including the special components that relate to trauma. The assessment progresses through the scene size-up, initial assessment, rapid trauma assessment (for the serious or critical patient) or the focused assessment and history, detailed physical exam (in rare cases), and finally, ongoing assessments.

During the scene size-up, you evaluate the scene to investigate and determine the mechanism of injury and, from that, identify an index of suspicion for specific injuries. You also analyze the potential hazards of the scene, including the need for body substance isolation procedures. You should search out and identify all patients. And, finally, you identify and summon all resources needed to manage the patients and scene.

In the initial assessment, you quickly apply spinal precautions and form a general patient impression and then determine the patient's mental status. Then, evaluate the patient's airway and breathing and perform any needed interventions (oxygen, oral or nasal airway or endotracheal intubation, and ventilation). Evaluate the circulation, control external hemorrhage, and, if hypovolemia and shock are possible, then initiate a large-bore IV. At the conclusion of the initial assessment, the patient is categorized as needing the rapid trauma assessment (emergency patients) or the focused trauma assessment.

During the rapid trauma assessment, you examine areas where significant injury is expected either from the mechanism of injury analysis or the initial assessment. It is also a time to examine the patient's chief and minor complaints, as time and priority permit. In general, during this assessment you should look in detail at the head, neck, chest, abdomen, and pelvis, as these are the areas likely to produce life-threatening injury. Take a quick set of vital signs and an abbreviated patient history. At the end of the rapid trauma assessment, decide the priority of the patient for transport. That decision is made by comparing the assessment findings against the trauma triage criteria used in your system.

The focused trauma assessment is used for the patient with limited mechanism of injury and expected, isolated, and moderate to minor injuries. During the focused assessment, you direct consideration to the likely injuries and the specific patient complaints. It usually concludes with slow transport to a nearby emergency department, or in some cases, treatment and release.

The detailed physical exam is a head-to-toe assessment of the patient while you search for signs and symptoms of injury. This procedure is useful for the unconscious patient for whom all other known or suspected life threats have been attended to, and it is then provided only during transport. However, portions of the techniques and process of the detailed assessment are used for elements of the initial and focused assessments.

During the ongoing assessment, you retake the vital signs, make a mental status assessment, reevaluate chief or serious patient complaints and significant signs of injury, and recheck any intervention you have performed. Perform an ongoing assessment every 5 minutes with seriously injured patients and every 15 minutes with other patients. Also perform the ongoing assessment after every major intervention or any sign that the patient's condition has changed or is changing.

5. Identify the importance of rapid recognition and treatment of shock in trauma patients. pp. 468–470

Shock is the transitional state between cardiovascular homeostasis and death. It develops rapidly in the presence of blood loss, respiratory compromise, and other problems. To be successful in combating this problem, you must recognize it early and employ aggressive and specific care. Recognition of shock is not at all easy as the body compensates for its effects by shrinking the vascular container, increasing peripheral vascular resistance, directing blood to only the most critical organs, and increasing heart rate. These actions are all to keep the body functioning and assure adequate perfusion. They make the recognition of early compensation for shock very difficult, however. Since shock in trauma is most commonly due to progressing blood loss, its rapid recognition followed by aggressive intervention and rapid transport are essential.

6. Identify and explain the value of the components of shock trauma resuscitation. pp. 470–472

The components of shock trauma resuscitation protect the spine, assure the patency of the airway, provide adequate ventilation, and support the circulatory system to maintain adequate perfusion.

The spine is protected from the moment that injury is suspected with manual immobilization of the head. A cervical collar is applied to support the spine, eventually the patient is secured to the long spine board, and then his head is secured (maintaining immobilization) to assure the spine remains immobile.

The airway must be maintained either by the patient who is alert and oriented and capable of maintaining his own airway or the patient is intubated to definitively protect the airway. Early intubation (intubation before the patient is in immediate need of it) is sometimes required as some physiologic conditions (airway burns or airway soft-tissue trauma) will become progressively worse, making later intubation more difficult or impossible or if vomiting and aspiration is a risk. If intubation cannot be accomplished, cricothyrotomy may be necessary.

Ventilation is employed for the patient who is not maintaining adequate air exchange on his own. If the patient has some respirations, overdrive ventilation is required and should be coordinated with the patient's attempts at respiration, if possible. Overdrive ventilation is of great value for the patient with flail chest, as it changes the dynamics of respiration and minimizes the paradoxical movement. It is also of special benefit with rib fractures but should be used with caution for patients with internal chest injury as it may make the pneumothorax and tension pneumothorax worse and may induce emboli in the patient with serious chest trauma. Oxygen should be administered at high-flow rate via a nonrebreather mask and oxygen saturation should be maintained at no less than 95 percent.

External hemorrhage must be controlled with direct pressure, elevation, pressure points, and, if absolutely necessary, with a tourniquet. Large-bore IVs should be introduced using non-restrictive administration sets and, preferably, lactated Ringer's solution. Fluid resuscitation should be at a keep-vein-open rate until the blood pressure drops to below 100 systolic; at that point, aggressive attempts should then be made to keep it above 90. Should the blood pressure fall to below 50 systolic, all attempts to infuse fluid rapidly should be used. Remember, however, that prehospital fluid resuscitation is generally restricted to a maximum of 3,000 mL of fluid. If necessary, titrate your fluid flow to assure you do not run out of solution before arriving at the emergency department.

7. Describe the special needs and assessment considerations when treating pediatric and geriatric trauma patients.
pp. 472–479

Pediatric patients are anatomically smaller than adults and present with several considerations that must be recognized as we provide prehospital emergency care. Their smaller size means that they have a greater body surface area with respect to total body mass and volume. This means injury to the skin, such as a burn, has greater consequences as the body has fewer resources to combat the fluid loss, body heat loss, and the infection commonly associated with severe burns. Children are also more prone to rapid heat loss and gain with unprotected exposure to the environment. Blood and fluid losses are also of consequence since these patients have smaller reserves to restore such losses. Their smaller size also determines how trauma will affect them. They often receive trauma higher on the anatomy than adults because of their lower height (as in pedestrian collisions), and their shorter arms and legs are less able to protect the trunk and head from trauma. The larger and more massive size of the head (proportionally) subjects it to a greater incidence of trauma. The bones at birth are mostly cartilaginous and very flexible; with time, these become calcified, stronger, and more rigid. This means, however, that during the early years the bones provide less protection for the brain and intrathoracic organs. These are the years in which the characteristic early childhood fracture, the greenstick fracture, is seen. Once seriously injured, children will generally compensate very well, often hiding the severity of the internal injuries. They also may not communicate their symptoms very effectively, and their vital signs are dynamic and change rapidly with age.

At the other end of the age spectrum, elderly patients pose some obstacles to assessment and care as well. Because they make up the fastest growing portion of the population, we must be more able to determine and respond to their special needs. These patients are subject to both the effects of aging and to the accumulating effects of chronic disease. Reduced reflexes dull their perceptions of the environment and make them more prone to trauma. Their highly calcified and brittle bones fracture more easily, sometimes with the stress of everyday activities, and heal poorly. Their brains occupy less of the cranium, making brain injuries more common. They have smaller cardiac reserves and less vibrant vascular systems, which means less tolerance of and poorer compensation for hypovolemia. Their systems are also more prone to disorders of hydration and more adversely affected by them. Their respiratory systems are, likewise, less compliant and have much smaller reserves. Finally, heat regulation is less dynamic and geriatric patients are more likely to suffer core temperature variations. Assessment of geriatric patients can be complicated by poor mentation on the patients' part and reduction in their ability to perceive pain.

8. Explain the importance of good communications with other personnel within the emergency medical services system. pp. 479–481

Good communication among the parties caring for the injury victim ensures that essential information is concisely and quickly communicated as patient care responsibilities are shifted from the First Responder, to the EMT, to the paramedic, to the flight crew, to the emergency nurse, and finally to the emergency physician. Any breakdown in communication along this chain can mean that vital information gained from assessment or regarding the care already given can be lost and the patient's potential for survival or recovery put at risk. Good communication also establishes our position and gains respect within the health care community and among the public at large. And, most importantly, our communication with the public helps to assure their confidence in our knowledge, our skills, our intent to serve patients, and our commitment to patient confidentiality.

9. Identify the benefits of helicopter use and list the criteria for establishing a landing zone. pp. 482–486

The helicopter has the ability to bypass traffic and transport the trauma patient directly from the scene of an incident to the trauma center at a speed roughly twice that of ground transport. Since the object of prehospital trauma care is to bring the patient to surgery quickly, the helicopter offers a great service to the trauma patient.

Landing zone criteria:
Flat surface
Debris-free
Obstruction-free—trees, utility lines, etc.
Free of ignition sources

Landing zone size:
60 × 60 feet—small helicopter
75 × 75 feet—medium helicopter
120 × 120 feet—large helicopter

10. Describe the preparation of a patient for air medical transport. pp. 486–487

The use of air medical transport for the trauma patient from the scene to a trauma center can significantly reduce transport time and save critical minutes of the "Golden Hour." A patient who will be flown should have the airway secured, at least one large-bore IV route established, and be completely and firmly immobilized. You should be prepared to give a rapid and thorough patient report when the flight crew arrives.

11. Identify the value of trauma care research and how it has impacted prehospital skills. pp. 487–488

Much of what we do in prehospital care has not been proven to make a difference in patient outcome. As we grow as a profession and medicine advances, we will be asked to justify those skills and modalities of care we use. That justification will only be accepted by the medical profession and society as a whole if it is borne out of scientific research. As we move into the 21st century, we must begin to research current and new drugs, techniques, and equipment to ensure they benefit our patients.

CASE STUDY REVIEW

Reread the case study on pages 445 and 446 in Paramedic Care: Trauma Emergencies *before reading the discussion below.*
The patient presented in this case study has the typical signs and symptoms of shock and is cared for with the aggressiveness required if shock resuscitation is to be successful.

Peter presents with the classic signs and symptoms of shock very early in assessment and care, suggesting that blood loss is rapid and already significant. The carotid pulse is rapid and weak, reflective of volume depletion and the heart's attempt to compensate with a rapid rate. The patient has a reduced level of consciousness, is not able to remember what happened, and is both anxious and combative. These signs reflect cerebral hypoxia. Breathing is also affected. Peter's breaths are shallow and rapid, thus less efficient than slower and deeper respirations. The absence of distal pulses suggests both reduced blood pressure and peripheral vasoconstriction. This is supported by the cool, clammy skin and capillary refill time of over 4 seconds (normal being less than 3 seconds). The pulse oximetry reading is low, reflecting poor oxygenation. It is surprising that a reading was obtained at all. In low-flow states, the oximeter often provides an erratic reading, if one can be obtained at all (suggesting low flow and very weak distal arterial pulsation).

This patient is certainly a candidate for rapid transport with aggressive shock care en route. Because of the entrapment, rapid transport is not an immediately available option and aggressive field care is employed. The aggressive care offered by Alex includes two IVs begun with 14- or 16-gauge short catheters. This will allow the greatest infusion rates. The catheters are connected to trauma tubing for the rapid infusion of crystalloids and, eventually, blood in the emergency department. Alex uses one 1,000 mL bag of lactated Ringer's solution and one of normal saline. The normal saline is hung because there is an incompatibility between blood and lactated Ringer's solution. This arrangement will allow the hospital to immediately infuse the blood through the saline line, if they wish to do so.

The PASG provides a double benefit in this patient scenario. The pressure of the garment over the dressings is an effective application of direct pressure and hemorrhage control. The garment also effectively supports the body's compensatory mechanisms against shock.

Alex awaits the arrival of the medical helicopter, probably because they are moments from arriving when Peter is extricated and transport to a pre-designated landing zone might increase the transfer time. It will be important for Alex to have this patient firmly secured to the spine board and the IV lines secured as well. The patient report must be abbreviated and specific to pertinent elements of Alex's initial, rapid trauma assessment and ongoing assessments because time is a precious element in this response and Peter's chances for survival. Pressure infusers are applied to the fluid bags by the flight team and pressurized to increase fluid flow. The flight crew's care benefits Peter because they have available and can administer O-negative blood, which helps replace lost plasma and red blood cells.

The only action on the part of the paramedic team that might have improved patient care would have been to draw blood at the scene and have a police officer transport it to the emergency department. This would allow the ED staff to type and crossmatch whole blood for the patient much earlier than would otherwise be possible. Instead, O-negative blood was given, which might not be the ideal blood type for this patient.

CONTENT SELF-EVALUATION

MULTIPLE CHOICE

_____ 1. The number of lives lost each year to trauma is:
  A. 78,000.
  B. 95,000.
  C. 110,000.
  D. 150,000.
  E. 210,000.

_____ 2. Injury prevention steps for EMS include which of the following?
  A. supporting pre-existing programs that support prevention
  B. acquainting the population with EMS
  C. alerting society to hazards
  D. performing home inspections
  E. all of the above

_____ 3. An EMS home inspection might examine for:
  A. hot water temperature.
  B. pool fencing.
  C. smoke detector battery levels.
  D. crib slat spacing.
  E. all of the above

_____ 4. Which of the following is a group especially at risk for trauma?
   A. young women
   B. young men
   C. the middle-age female
   D. the middle age male
   E. elderly women

_____ 5. The dispatch information is likely to provide you with which of the following?
   A. the location of the incident
   B. any suspected scene hazards
   C. any suspected danger of violence
   D. other units responding
   E. all of the above

_____ 6. When approaching a scene of suspected violence, you should:
   A. enter the scene immediately.
   B. enter the scene if it seems calm.
   C. enter the scene if the police are there.
   D. enter the scene if you are told it is safe by the police.
   E. none of the above

_____ 7. What level of body substance isolation will you employ at all trauma scenes?
   A. gloves
   B. goggles
   C. gloves and goggles
   D. gown
   E. gloves and gown

_____ 8. The analysis of the mechanism of injury provides you with which item of patient information that is used during the initial and rapid trauma assessments?
   A. the number of patients
   B. the type of impact
   C. the resources needed
   D. the index of suspicion
   E. the hazards at the scene

_____ 9. Once you identify the type and nature of a hazardous material, attempt to enter the scene and remove the patient if there is any danger present.
   A. True
   B. False

_____ 10. The risk of contamination and resultant disease from contact with body substances is greater for you than for your patient.
   A. True
   B. False

_____ 11. In the case where you are assessing several patients, some with hemorrhage, you should:
   A. use one glove set per patient
   B. use one glove set per patient contact
   C. use one set of gloves for all patient contacts
   D. wash your hands (with gloves on) between contacts
   E. none of the above

_____ 12. If you arrive at a scene where a patient is covered with blood and has it spurting from an open facial wound, appropriate BSI is:
   A. gloves.
   B. gloves and goggles.
   C. gloves and gown.
   D. gloves and mask.
   E. gloves, goggles, mask, and gown.

_____ 13. Air medical service should be summoned for any serious trauma scene if transport time will exceed:
   A. 15 minutes.
   B. 15 to 20 minutes.
   C. 20 to 30 minutes.
   D. 30 to 40 minutes.
   E. 1 hour.

_____ 14. The reason for calling in additional resources before arriving at the patient's side is to ensure the needed resources arrive in a timely manner.
   A. True
   B. False

_____ 15. Which of the following is an element of the initial assessment?
A. spinal precautions
B. a general patient impression
C. mental status evaluation
D. airway maintenance
E. all of the above

_____ 16. Which of the following injury mechanisms would require spinal precautions?
A. severe flexion/extension
B. severe lateral bending
C. severe distraction
D. severe axial loading
E. all of the above

_____ 17. The general impression of the patient is a difficult impression to make accurately early in a paramedic's career.
A. True
B. False

_____ 18. If your impression of a patient conflicts with the seriousness of potential injuries suggested by the mechanism of injury analysis, you should:
A. act according to your general impression.
B. reanalyze the mechanism of injury analysis.
C. determine vital signs and then determine patient priority.
D. suspect the worst of the indicators is correct and act accordingly.
E. not worry as the patient's true condition will become more evident with time.

_____ 19. The "A" of the AVPU mnemonic stands for:
A. altered mental status.
B. alert.
C. adjusted to time.
D. accurate.
E. attitude.

_____ 20. Which is the order in which levels of orientation are lost?
A. time, persons, place
B. time, place, persons
C. persons, place, time
D. persons, time, place
E. place, persons, time

_____ 21. The movement by the patient away from a painful stimulus is termed:
A. purposeful.
B. purposeless.
C. decorticate posturing.
D. decerebrate posturing.
E. painful.

_____ 22. The movement by the patient to a position of muscular extension with the elbows flexing is termed:
A. purposeful.
B. purposeless.
C. decorticate posturing.
D. decerebrate posturing.
E. painful.

_____ 23. It is easy to determine that the airway of a conscious and alert patient is patent when he can speak clearly in normal sentences.
A. True
B. False

_____ 24. If the patient does not have a gag reflex, when should you intubate him?
A. at the end of the assessment
B. once there are signs of emesis
C. immediately
D. delay intubation but insert an oral airway
E. none of the above

_____ 25. If you find it necessary to ventilate a patient, you should do so at a rate of:
A. 10 to 16 per minute.
B. 12 to 20 per minute.
C. 12 to 24 per minute.
D. 16 to 30 per minute.
E. 30 to 40 per minute.

_____ 26. Capillary refill is no longer of value in the assessment of the pediatric patient.
    A. True
    B. False

_____ 27. Which of the following will affect the rate of capillary refill in the adult patient?
    A. smoking
    B. low ambient temperatures
    C. pre-existing disease
    D. use of certain medications
    E. all of the above

_____ 28. A weak, thready pulse suggests shock compensation.
    A. True
    B. False

_____ 29. In people with pigmented skin, examine for discoloration of the:
    A. lips.
    B. sclera.
    C. palms.
    D. soles of the feet.
    E. all of the above

_____ 30. Hyperresonance on percussion of the chest suggests:
    A. blood accumulation.
    B. fluid accumulation.
    C. air.
    D. air under pressure.
    E. both C and D

_____ 31. The detailed physical exam is used rarely in prehospital trauma care.
    A. True
    B. False

_____ 32. When one eye is shaded, the opposite pupil should:
    A. remain as it is.
    B. dilate briskly.
    C. dilate slowly.
    D. constrict briskly.
    E. constrict slowly.

_____ 33. You notice flat jugular veins in the supine patient. This suggests:
    A. tension pneumothorax.
    B. pericardial tamponade.
    C. a normotensive patient.
    D. a hypovolemic patient.
    E. infection.

_____ 34. Allergies to which of the following drugs may be important in the treatment of the trauma patient?
    A. "caine" drugs
    B. antibiotics
    C. tetanus toxoid
    D. analgesics
    E. all of the above

_____ 35. Which of the following is NOT indicative of shock compensation?
    A. a falling blood pressure
    B. an increasing pulse rate
    C. a decreasing level of consciousness
    D. a decreasing pulse strength
    E. cool and clammy skin

_____ 36. Transport decisions for serious trauma patients are determined by the use of:
    A. trauma score.
    B. Glasgow Coma Scale score.
    C. trauma triage criteria.
    D. vital signs.
    E. helicopter availability.

_____ 37. A trauma patient is breathing at 12 times per minute, has normal respiratory expansion, a blood pressure of 96 systolic, delayed capillary refill of 4 seconds, and a Glasgow Coma Scale score of 10. What should you report as the trauma score to medical control?
    A. 7
    B. 9
    C. 10
    D. 11
    E. 15

_____ 38. The ongoing assessment should be performed every 15 minutes on the seriously injured trauma patient.
   A. True
   B. False

_____ 39. Which of the following terms refers to the reduction of fluid volume within the cardiovascular system?
   A. hypovolemia
   B. hypoperfusion
   C. hypotension
   D. anemia
   E. mimesis

_____ 40. Which of the following terms refers to a low blood pressure?
   A. hypovolemia
   B. hypoperfusion
   C. hypotension
   D. anemia
   E. none of the above

_____ 41. Normally, the prehospital infusion of crystalloids in the resuscitation of a shock patient should be limited to:
   A. 500 mL.
   B. 1,000 mL.
   C. 2,000 mL.
   D. 3,000 mL.
   E. 5,000 mL.

_____ 42. Hypothermia is a serious complication of shock that compromises the patient's clotting mechanisms.
   A. True
   B. False

_____ 43. What percentage of trauma responses are for non-critical cases?
   A. 30 percent
   B. 50 percent
   C. 65 percent
   D. 80 percent
   E. 95 percent

_____ 44. Which of the following statements is NOT true regarding the pediatric patient as compared to the adult patient?
   A. The child's surface area to volume ratio is greater.
   B. The child's organs are closer together.
   C. The child's airway is smaller.
   D. The child compensates for blood loss poorly.
   E. The child's skeletal components are more flexible.

_____ 45. The healthy pediatric patient may compensate for blood loss up to what percentage?
   A. 25 percent
   B. 35 percent
   C. 45 percent
   D. 50 percent
   E. 60 percent

_____ 46. Which of the following is NOT true regarding pediatric vital signs as the child ages?
   A. The temperature rises.
   B. The pulse rate decreases.
   C. The tidal volume increases.
   D. The blood pressure increases.
   E. The respirations slow.

_____ 47. The oral airway should be inserted by rotating it 180 degrees during insertion for the pediatric patient.
   A. True
   B. False

_____ 48. The additional IV access site not commonly used for the adult but available for the pediatric patient is the:
   A. subclavian vein.
   B. intraosseous site.
   C. antecubital fossa.
   D. popliteal vein.
   E. scalp vein.

49. The recommended size of the initial fluid bolus for a pediatric trauma patient is:
  A. 100 mL.
  B. 250 mL.
  C. 20 mL/kg.
  D. 60 mL/kg.
  E. 80 mL/kg.

50. Which is the fastest growing group of EMS patients?
  A. the elderly
  B. pediatric patients
  C. young males
  D. young females
  E. middle-aged patients

51. Which of the following statements is NOT true regarding elderly patients?
  A. They have a lower pain tolerance.
  B. Renal function is decreased.
  C. Brain mass and volume are decreased.
  D. Lung function is decreased.
  E. Cardiac stroke volume is decreased.

52. Because of chronic and pre-existing diseases, geriatric patients move into which of these conditions more quickly than healthy adults?
  A. shock compensation
  B. decompensated shock
  C. irreversible shock
  D. death
  E. all of the above

53. Assessment of the geriatric patient is often difficult because the underlying problem that leads the patient to call EMS is often masked or confused by signs and symptoms of pre-existing disease.
  A. True
  B. False

54. Key elements of the oral patient care report include all of the following EXCEPT:
  A. mechanism of injury.
  B. response times.
  C. results of assessment.
  D. interventions.
  E. results of interventions.

55. Which of the following is NOT appropriate handling of contaminated material during or after the trauma call?
  A. recapping needles
  B. placing needles in a sharps container
  C. wearing BSI during equipment cleaning
  D. scanning the scene for contaminated supplies
  E. placing soiled linen in biohazard bags

56. Which of the following is NOT an advantage to air medical transport of the trauma patient?
  A. The helicopter travels at very high speeds
  B. The helicopter provides a superior working environment
  C. The helicopter can bypass traffic congestion
  D. The helicopter can travel is a straight line
  E. none of the above

57. The landing zone for a medium-sized helicopter should be at least:
  A. 25 by 25 feet.
  B. 40 by 40 feet.
  C. 60 by 60 feet.
  D. 75 by 75 feet.
  E. 120 by 120 feet.

58. The lights illuminating the landing zone should shine upward to help the pilot locate the center of the zone.
  A. True
  B. False

_____ **59.** Rising in the helicopter is likely to cause all of the following conditions to worsen EXCEPT:
  A. COPD.
  B. hypovolemia.
  C. tension pneumothorax.
  D. asthma.
  E. endotracheal tube cuff pressure.

_____ **60.** The environment inside a helicopter often makes it difficult to:
  A. hear breath sounds.
  B. feel a pulse.
  C. communicate with the patient.
  D. intubate the patient.
  E. all of the above

SPECIAL PROJECT

Crossword Puzzle

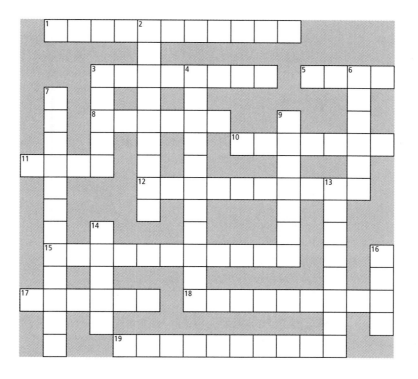

Across
1. Referring to the regulation of the cardiovascular system
3. An open wound caused by a scraping trauma
5. The outermost layer of the meninges
8. The fluid portion of the blood
10. The type of energy related to motion
11. Ionizing radiation that can penetrate only superficial layers of clothing or the skin
12. The transitional region of the bone between the diaphysis and the epiphysis
15. The collapse of the alveoli
17. The smaller of the bones of the lower leg
18. A closed soft-tissue wound
19. An open wound which may be gaping and jagged

Down
2. A surface area of the body controlled by one peripheral nerve root
3. The weakest form of ionizing radiation
4. The "fight-or-flight" nervous system
6. The lateral bone of the forearm
7. Increase in velocity
9. Biological catalysts which help break down food
13. A smooth form of laceration
14. The bone of the thigh
16. The medial bone of the forearm

TRAUMA EMERGENCIES
Content Review

CONTENT SELF-EVALUATION

Chapter 1: Trauma and Trauma Systems

_____ 1. Trauma accounts for about what death toll each year?
- A. 100,000 deaths
- B. 150,000 deaths
- C. 200,000 deaths
- D. 250,000 deaths
- E. 400,000 deaths

_____ 2. Serious life-threatening injury occurs in about 30 percent of all trauma.
- A. True
- B. False

_____ 3. Trauma care is predicated on the principle that serious trauma is a(n):
- A. noncomplex medical problem.
- B. surgical disease.
- C. EMT-B concern.
- D. circumstance best cared for by emergency physicians.
- E. Level I trauma center concern.

_____ 4. A Level III trauma center is a(n):
- A. community hospital.
- B. teaching hospital.
- C. emergency department with 24-hour service.
- D. non-emergency health care facility.
- E. regional center.

_____ 5. The guidelines that help determine the need of a trauma patient for the services of the trauma center are called the:
- A. mechanism of injury.
- B. index of suspicion.
- C. trauma triage criteria.
- D. surgical guidelines.
- E. Golden Hour.

_____ 6. The result of the analysis of the mechanism of injury is the:
- A. Golden Hour concept.
- B. kinetic analysis of the trauma.
- C. scene size-up.
- D. index of suspicion.
- E. expected injury algorithm.

_____ 7. The major advantage to helicopter transport of the trauma patient is that helicopters travel much faster than ground units and in a straight line.
- A. True
- B. False

_____ 8. Because paramedics are usually at the side of seriously injured patients so quickly, the signs and symptoms of serious injury and shock will be apparent.
- A. True
- B. False

_____ 9. One of the most effective methods of reducing trauma morbidity and mortality is through injury prevention programs.
   A. True
   B. False

_____ 10. Which of the following indicates a trauma patient's need for immediate transport to a trauma center?
   A. systolic blood pressure less than 90 mmHg
   B. flail chest
   C. ejection from a vehicle
   D. fall from greater than 3 times the victim's height
   E. all of the above

Chapter 2: Blunt Trauma

_____ 11. The capacity to do work is termed:
   A. kinetics.   D. inertia.
   B. velocity.   E. momentum.
   C. energy.

_____ 12. Blunt trauma does not cause injury beneath the skin.
   A. True
   B. False

_____ 13. Auto collisions account for about what number of deaths each year?
   A. 23,000   D. 50,000
   B. 38,000   E. 100,000
   C. 44,000

_____ 14. Place the events of an auto collision in the order in which they occur.
   A. body collision, vehicle collision, organ collision, secondary collisions
   B. organ collision, vehicle collision, body collision, secondary collisions
   C. vehicle collision, secondary collisions, body collision, organ collision
   D. vehicle collision, body collision, organ collision, secondary collisions
   E. body collision, vehicle collision, secondary collisions, organ collision

_____ 15. Which of the following have played a substantial role in reducing highway collision related deaths?
   A. shoulder belts   D. child seats
   B. passenger airbags   E. all of the above
   C. driver airbags

_____ 16. The seat belt is very effective at reducing injuries related to intrusion into the auto passenger compartment.
   A. True
   B. False

_____ 17. Which of the following are injuries that airbag inflation may cause?
   A. hand injuries   D. nasal fractures
   B. finger injuries   E. all of the above
   C. facial injuries

_____ 18. The up-and-over pathway is most commonly associated with which auto collision type?
   A. lateral   D. rear-end
   B. rotational   E. rollover
   C. frontal

_____ 19. When analyzing the frontal impact injury mechanism, the paramedic should assign a higher index of suspicion for serious life-threatening injury than with other types of impacts.
   A. True
   B. False

_____ 20. The type of injury most commonly associated with the rear-end impact is:
   A. head injury.
   B. pelvic injury.
   C. neck injury.
   D. foot fracture.
   E. abdominal injury.

_____ 21. When you encounter the intoxicated patient, the mechanism of injury analysis becomes even more important.
   A. True
   B. False

_____ 22. The helmet reduces the incidence of head injury by about what percent?
   A. 25
   B. 35
   C. 50
   D. 65
   E. 80

_____ 23. In the auto/adult pedestrian collision, you would expect the victim to turn away from the impact.
   A. True
   B. False

_____ 24. A victim standing and facing the epicenter of a blast is more likely to sustain serious injury than the victim lying on the ground with his feet toward the blast epicenter.
   A. True
   B. False

_____ 25. Shrapnel are small, arrow-like objects within a bomb casing that extend its injury potential and range.
   A. True
   B. False

_____ 26. Which of the following are primary blast injuries?
   A. heat injuries
   B. pressure injuries
   C. projectile injuries
   D. injuries caused by structural collapse
   E. both A and B

_____ 27. The closer a victim was to the epicenter of a blast, the higher should be the paramedic's index of suspicion for more serious injuries.
   A. True
   B. False

_____ 28. Ear injuries associated with an explosion, even those affecting as much as one-third of the eardrum with a tear, may improve with time.
   A. True
   B. False

_____ 29. In the terms of physics, a fall is nothing more than the release of stored gravitational energy.
   A. True
   B. False

_____ 30. Sports injuries are frequently associated with the mechanism of:
   A. compression.
   B. extension/flexion.
   C. compression/distraction.
   D. rotation.
   E. all of the above

Chapter 3: Penetrating Trauma

_____ 31. An object that weighs twice as much as another object traveling at the same speed has:
   A. twice the kinetic energy.
   B. three times the kinetic energy.
   C. four times the kinetic energy.
   D. five times the kinetic energy.
   E. six times the kinetic energy.

_____ 32. Wounds from a handgun are two to four times more lethal than those from a rifle.
   A. True
   B. False

_____ 33. The diameter of a projectile is its:
   A. caliber.
   B. profile.
   C. drag.
   D. yaw.
   E. expansion factor.

_____ 34. Which of the following is a characteristic of a handgun bullet in contrast to a rifle bullet?
   A. It is a heavier projectile.
   B. It travels at a greater velocity.
   C. It has a blunter shape.
   D. It is more likely to fragment.
   E. all of the above

_____ 35. With low-velocity penetrating objects, the extent of injury is easy to determine because the depth of entry and the pathway are easy to determine.
   A. True
   B. False

_____ 36. Which element of the projectile injury process describes the region filled with air and tissue debris after the bullet has passed?
   A. direct injury
   B. pressure wave
   C. temporary cavity
   D. permanent cavity
   E. zone of injury

_____ 37. The tissue structures that are very dense and usually sustain significant damage with the passage of a projectile are the:
   A. solid organs.
   B. hollow organs.
   C. connective tissue.
   D. bones.
   E. lungs.

_____ 38. The tissue structures that are very resilient and usually sustain the smallest amount of damage associated with the passage of a projectile are the:
   A. solid organs.
   B. hollow organs.
   C. connective tissue.
   D. bones.
   E. lungs.

_____ 39. The abdominal organ rather tolerant to the passage of a projectile is the:
   A. bowel.
   B. liver.
   C. spleen.
   D. kidneys.
   E. pancreas.

_____ 40. The impact of a bullet with the ribs may induce an explosive energy exchange that injures the surrounding tissue with numerous bony fragments.
   A. True
   B. False

_____ 41. A penetrating wound to the area of the rib margin should be suspected of involving the:
   A. spleen or liver.
   B. kidneys.
   C. abdominal and thoracic organs.
   D. left, right, or both lung fields.
   E. all of the above

_____ 42. Generally, powder burns and tattooing around the entrance wound suggest use of a:
  A. gun at close range.
  B. high-powered rifle.
  C. handgun.
  D. black powder weapon.
  E. shotgun.

_____ 43. Which of the following is frequently associated with an exit wound?
  A. tattooing
  B. a small ridge of discoloration around the wound
  C. a blown-out appearance
  D. subcutaneous emphysema
  E. propellant residue on the surrounding tissue

_____ 44. The exit wound is usually more likely to reflect the actual damaging potential of the projectile.
  A. True
  B. False

_____ 45. A relatively small bullet wound to the chest is all that is necessary to produce an open pneumothorax.
  A. True
  B. False

Chapter 4: Hemorrhage and Shock

_____ 46. Which of the following, through hormones, most specifically increases the heart rate?
  A. the autonomic nervous system
  B. the sympathetic nervous system
  C. the parasympathetic nervous system
  D. the somatic nervous system
  E. the voluntary nervous system

_____ 47. Which of the following affects the stroke volume of the heart?
  A. preload
  B. afterload
  C. cardiac contractility
  D. ventricular filling
  E. all of the above

_____ 48. The muscular layer controlling the lumen of a vessel is the:
  A. tunica adventicia.
  B. tunica media.
  C. tunica intima.
  D. the escarpment.
  E. none of the above

_____ 49. Approximately what volume of the body's blood is contained within the capillaries?
  A. 7%
  B. 13%
  C. 64%
  D. 23%
  E. 45%

_____ 50. The red blood cells account for what percentage of the total blood volume?
  A. 45%
  B. 78%
  C. 86%
  D. 92%
  E. 99%

_____ 51. Which of the following types of hemorrhage is characterized by slow-oozing bright red blood?
  A. capillary bleeding
  B. venous bleeding
  C. arterial bleeding
  D. both A and C
  E. none of the above

_____ 52. Which of the following is the phase of clotting in which smooth muscle contracts?
  A. intrinsic phase
  B. vascular phase
  C. platelet phase
  D. coagulation phase
  E. aggregation phase

_____ 53. Blood vessels that are lacerated longitudinally generally do not bleed very severely or for very long.
  A. True
  B. False

_____ 54. Which of the following is likely to adversely affect the clotting process?
  A. aggressive fluid resuscitation
  B. hypothermia
  C. movement at the site of injury
  D. drugs such as aspirin
  E. all of the above

_____ 55. Fractures of the tibia or humerus can account for a blood loss of:
  A. less than 500 mL.
  B. from 500 to 750 mL.
  C. up to 1,500 mL.
  D. from 1,500 to 2,000 mL.
  E. in excess of 2,000 mL.

_____ 56. In which stage of hemorrhage does the patient first display ineffective respiration?
  A. the first stage
  B. the second stage
  C. the third stage
  D. the fourth stage
  E. the terminal stage

_____ 57. The female in late pregnancy is likely to have a blood volume that is:
  A. much less than normal.
  B. slightly less than normal.
  C. slightly greater than normal.
  D. much greater than normal.
  E. normal.

_____ 58. A fast and weak pulse may be the first indication of developing shock in the trauma patient.
  A. True
  B. False

_____ 59. Large hematomas can account for a blood loss of:
  A. up to 500 mL.
  B. from 500 to 750 mL.
  C. up to 1,500 mL.
  D. from 1,500 to 2,000 mL.
  E. in excess of 2,000 mL.

_____ 60. Frank blood in the stool is called:
  A. hemoptysis.
  B. melena.
  C. hematuria.
  D. hematochezia.
  E. hematemesis.

_____ 61. For the patient in compensated shock, you should perform an ongoing assessment:
  A. every 5 minutes.
  B. every 15 minutes.
  C. after every major intervention.
  D. after noting any change in signs or symptoms.
  E. all except B

_____ 62. The systolic blood pressure reflects the:
  A. strength of cardiac output.
  B. volume of cardiac output.
  C. state of peripheral vascular resistance.
  D. state of arteriole constriction.
  E. both A and B

_____ 63. The brain and heart can survive and perform well with blood flowing through them from 5 to 20 percent of the time.
  A. True
  B. False

_____ 64. Which of the following is a result of sympathetic nervous system stimulation?
A. increased heart rate
B. increased peripheral vascular resistance
C. increased cardiac contractility
D. skeletal muscle vasodilation
E. all of the above

_____ 65. Which of the following is a catecholamine?
A. glucagon
B. insulin
C. norepinephrine
D. adrenocorticotropic hormone
E. erythropoietin

_____ 66. Which of the following is a potent system vasoconstrictor?
A. antidiuretic hormone
B. angiotensin II
C. aldosterone
D. epinephrine
E. erythropoietin

_____ 67. The opening of post-capillary sphincters and the resulting release of potassium, acids, and hypoxic blood is called:
A. ischemia.
B. rouleaux.
C. washout.
D. hydrostatic release.
E. none of the above

_____ 68. During which stage of shock is it difficult to determine if the patient is suffering from the effects of hypovolemia?
A. compensatory
B. decompensatory
C. irreversible
D. hypovolemic
E. cardiogenic

_____ 69. Which of the following does NOT first occur during the decompensated stage of shock?
A. Pulses become unpalpable.
B. Respirations slow or cease.
C. Blood pressure decreases precipitously.
D. The skin becomes cool and clammy.
E. The patient becomes unconscious.

_____ 70. Under which of the following shock types would septic shock fall?
A. hypovolemic
B. distributive
C. obstructive
D. cardiogenic
E. respiratory

_____ 71. Under which of the following shock types would pericardial tamponade fall?
A. hypovolemic
B. distributive
C. obstructive
D. cardiogenic
E. respiratory

_____ 72. The color, temperature, and general appearance of the skin can indicate shock before there are changes in the blood pressure.
A. True
B. False

_____ 73. In the normovolemic patient the jugular veins should be full when the patient is supine.
A. True
B. False

_____ 74. Which of the following will permit the least fluid flow through a catheter?
A. short length, small lumen
B. short length, large lumen
C. long length, small lumen
D. long length, large lumen
E. large lumen and either long or short length

_____ 75. The preferred electrolyte solution for the patient who is losing blood is:
A. normal saline.
B. dextrose 5 percent in water.
C. lactated Ringer's solution.
D. hypertonic saline.
E. hypotonic saline.

Chapter 5: Soft-Tissue Trauma

_____ 76. Which of the following glands secrete a waxy substance?
A. sudoriferous glands
B. sebaceous glands
C. subcutaneous glands
D. adrenal glands
E. pituitary glands

_____ 77. The layer of skin that is made up of mostly dead cells and provides the waterproof envelope that contains the body is the:
A. dermis.
B. subcutaneous layer.
C. epidermis.
D. sebum.
E. corium.

_____ 78. Identify the layers of the arteries and veins in order from exterior to interior.
A. intima, media, adventitia
B. media, intima, adventitia
C. adventitia, intima, media
D. adventitia, media, intima
E. intima, adventitia, media

_____ 79. The blood vessels that have a wall only one cell thick are the:
A. arteries.
B. arterioles.
C. capillaries.
D. venules.
E. veins.

_____ 80. In the limbs, fascia define compartments with relatively fixed volumes.
A. True
B. False

_____ 81. Lacerations perpendicular to skin tension lines will cause the wound to gape.
A. True
B. False

_____ 82. The wound type characterized by a collection of blood under the skin is the:
A. abrasion.
B. contusion.
C. laceration.
D. hematoma.
E. avulsion.

_____ 83. The wound type characterized by a deep wound whose opening closes after injury is the:
A. abrasion.
B. contusion.
C. laceration.
D. hematoma.
E. puncture.

_____ 84. Prolonged crush injury (crush syndrome) permits the accumulation of:
A. myoglobin.
B. potassium.
C. lactic acid.
D. uric acid.
E. all of the above

_____ 85. A likely cause of an avulsion is a(n):
A. animal bite.
B. severe glancing blow to the scalp.
C. machinery accident.
D. degloving injury.
E. all of the above

_____ 86. The natural ability of the body to halt blood loss is:
A. anemia.
B. homeostasis.
C. hemostasis.
D. coagulation.
E. metabolism.

87. Most blood vessels, when cut cleanly, will withdraw and constrict, limiting the rate of hemorrhage.
   A. True
   B. False

88. The cells that attack invading pathogens directly through an antibody response are:
   A. macrophages.
   B. lymphocytes.
   C. chemotactic factors.
   D. granulocytes.
   E. both A and D

89. The stage of the healing process in which skin cells regenerate to restore a uniform layer of skin cells along the wound border is:
   A. inflammation.
   B. epithelialization.
   C. neovascularization.
   D. collagen synthesis.
   E. none of the above

90. The stage of the healing process in which capillaries grow to perfuse the healing tissue is:
   A. inflammation.
   B. epithelialization.
   C. neovascularization.
   D. collagen synthesis.
   E. none of the above

91. Which of the following is a soft-tissue wound infection risk factor?
   A. HIV
   B. smoking
   C. avulsion
   D. COPD
   E. all of the above

92. The booster for tetanus is effective for:
   A. 1 year.
   B. 2 to 4 years.
   C. 5 years.
   D. 10 years.
   E. 25 years.

93. Which of the following can interfere with normal clotting?
   A. aspirin
   B. heparin
   C. TPA
   D. penicillin
   E. all of the above

94. The excessive growth of scar tissue beyond the boundaries of the wound is:
   A. hypertrophic scar formation.
   B. keloid scar formation.
   C. anatropic scar formation.
   D. residual scar formation.
   E. reactive scar formation.

95. The patient is not likely to experience pressure injury, even when immobilized for a lengthy period on a long spine board, PASG, or rigid splint.
   A. True
   B. False

96. The process of actual tissue death is:
   A. necrosis.
   B. ischemia.
   C. rhabdomyolysis.
   D. gangrene.
   E. mitosis.

97. Most dressings used in prehospital emergency care are sterile, nonocclusive, nonadherent, absorbent dressings.
   A. True
   B. False

98. The type of dressing that promotes clot development is:
   A. adherent.
   B. nonadherent.
   C. absorbent.
   D. occlusive.
   E. nonocclusive.

_____ 99. The type of bandage that has limited stretch and conforms well to the body contours is the:
   A. elastic bandage.
   B. self-adherent roller bandage.
   C. gauze bandage.
   D. adhesive bandage.
   E. none of the above

_____ 100. As a minimum, how long should you maintain pressure point pressure when trying to control hemorrhage?
   A. 2 minutes
   B. 4 minutes
   C. 6 minutes
   D. 8 minutes
   E. 10 minutes

_____ 101. The dangers of a tourniquet include:
   A. increased hemorrhage if pressure is not sufficient.
   B. possible loss of limb.
   C. accumulation of toxins in the limb.
   D. tissue damage beneath the tourniquet.
   E. all of the above

_____ 102. The restoration of circulation once a tourniquet is released may cause all of the following EXCEPT:
   A. emboli.
   B. hypovolemia.
   C. lethal dysrhythmias.
   D. massive vasoconstriction.
   E. renal failure.

_____ 103. You should remove gross contamination from a wound if you can do so quickly and without further injury.
   A. True
   B. False

_____ 104. Scalp hemorrhage is rarely severe or difficult to control.
   A. True
   B. False

_____ 105. The ideal position for splinting a limb is halfway between extension and flexion and is called the:
   A. anatomic position.
   B. physiologic position.
   C. neutral position.
   D. position of function.
   E. recovery position.

_____ 106. The recommended procedure for packaging an amputated part for transport includes:
   A. packing it in ice.
   B. keeping it at body temperature.
   C. keeping it dry and cool.
   D. keeping it wet and cool.
   E. freezing if immediately.

_____ 107. Most all patients of crush syndrome can be identified before extrication is complete.
   A. True
   B. False

_____ 108. Lactated Ringer's solution is recommended for the patient with crush syndrome since it replaces the fluids lost due to the injury.
   A. True
   B. False

_____ 109. With compartment syndrome, motor and sensory function are frequently normal.
   A. True
   B. False

_____ 110. A wound involving which of the following requires transport?
   A. nerves
   B. blood vessels
   C. tendons
   D. ligaments
   E. all of the above

Chapter 6: Burns

_____ 111. The incidence of burn injury has been on the increase over the past decade.
A. True
B. False

_____ 112. The layer of skin with capillary beds and sensory nerve endings is the:
A. dermis.
B. subcutaneous layer.
C. epidermis.
D. sebum.
E. corium.

_____ 113. Which of the following is NOT a function of the skin?
A. protecting the body from bacterial infection
B. aiding in temperature regulation
C. permitting joint movement
D. encouraging fluid loss in cold weather
E. accommodating body movement

_____ 114. Place the following phases of the body's burn response in the order in which they would be expected to occur.
A. emergent, fluid shift, hypermetabolic, resolution
B. fluid shift, hypermetabolic, resolution, emergent
C. fluid shift, resolution, emergent, hypermetabolic
D. hypermetabolic, fluid shift, emergent, resolution
E. emergent, resolution, hypermetabolic, fluid shift

_____ 115. The area of a burn that is characterized by reduced blood flow is generally the zone of:
A. hyperemia.
B. denaturing.
C. stasis.
D. coagulation.
E. most resistance.

_____ 116. Which of the following skin types has the least resistance to the passage of electrical current?
A. mucous membranes
B. wet skin
C. calluses
D. the skin on the inside of the arm
E. the skin on the inside of the thigh

_____ 117. Electrical arc or flash burns may be hot enough to vaporize body tissue.
A. True
B. False

_____ 118. Burns due to strong acids are likely to be less deep than burns due to strong alkalis because they produce liquefaction necrosis.
A. True
B. False

_____ 119. Which of the following radiation types is least powerful?
A. neutron
B. alpha
C. gamma
D. beta
E. delta

_____ 120. As radiation exposure increases, the signs of exposure become more evident and occur sooner.
A. True
B. False

_____ 121. Carbon monoxide has an affinity for hemoglobin that is how many times greater than oxygen has?
A. 10
B. 100
C. 200
D. 250
E. 325

_____ 122. Thermal airway burns occur more frequently than toxic inhalation injuries.
     A. True
     B. False

_____ 123. The burn characterized by erythema and pain only is the:
     A. superficial burn.   **D.** electrical burn.
     B. partial-thickness burn.   **E.** chemical burn.
     C. full-thickness burn.

_____ 124. The burn characterized by discoloration and lack of pain is the:
     A. superficial burn.   **D.** electrical burn.
     B. partial-thickness burn.   **E.** chemical burn.
     C. full-thickness burn.

_____ 125. A child patient has received burns to the entire anterior chest and to the entire left upper extremity circumferentially. Based on the rule of nines, what is the percentage of body surface area (BSA) involved?
     A. 9%   **D.** 36%
     B. 18%   **E.** 48%
     C. 27%

_____ 126. An adult patient receives burns to his entire head and neck and upper back. Based on the rule of nines, what is the percentage of BSA involved?
     A. 9%   **D.** 19%
     B. 10%   **E.** 27%
     C. 18%

_____ 127. Which of the following is a systemic complication that you should suspect with all serious burns?
     A. organ failure   **D.** complications caused by advancing age
     B. hypovolemia   **E.** all of the above
     C. infection

_____ 128. Once the suspected inhalation injury patient displays any signs of airway restriction, intubation should not be attempted as it will traumatize the airway tissue, increase swelling and further restrict the airway.
     A. True
     B. False

_____ 129. High-flow oxygen (100%) will reduce the half-life of carbon monoxide in the blood by up to two-thirds.
     A. True
     B. False

_____ 130. The patient you are attending has her entire left lower extremity seriously burned. The leg and foot are very painful and reddened while the thigh is relatively painless and a dark red color. What percentage of the BSA and burn depth would you assign this patient?
     A. 18 percent full-thickness burn
     B. 18 percent partial-thickness burn
     C. 9 percent full-thickness burn
     D. 9 percent partial-thickness burn
     E. 9 percent partial-thickness and 9 percent full-thickness burn

_____ 131. Your assessment reveals a burn patient with partial-thickness burns to 27 percent of the body. What classification of burn severity would you assign her?
     A. minor   **D.** critical
     B. moderate   **E.** none of the above
     C. serious

_____ 132. Your assessment reveals a burn patient with superficial burns to more than half the body. What classification of burn severity would you assign her?
A. minor
B. moderate
C. serious
D. critical
E. none of the above

_____ 133. Your assessment reveals a burn patient with partial-thickness burns to the face, though you have ruled out inhalation injury. What classification of burn severity would you assign her?
A. minor
B. moderate
C. serious
D. critical
E. none of the above

_____ 134. Which of the following burns would NOT be considered a critical burn?
A. a circumferential third-degree burn to the chest
B. superficial facial burns with sooty residue
C. 10 percent superficial and partial-thickness burns
D. full-thickness burns to the elbow and hand
E. 25 percent partial-thickness burns in the geriatric patient

_____ 135. Local and minor burns (superficial and partial-thickness) may be cared for with:
A. direct pressure.
B. cool water immersion.
C. prolonged application of ice.
D. warm water immersion.
E. A and D

_____ 136. In general, moderate to severe burns should be cared for with:
A. moist occlusive dressings.
B. dry sterile dressings.
C. cool water immersion.
D. plastic wrap covered by a soft dressing.
E. warm water immersion.

_____ 137. Nonadherent padding should be placed between full-thickness burns of the fingers and toes to prevent adhesion and damage when they are separated.
A. True
B. False

_____ 138. Even though there are no other intravenous sites available on a patient, you should not introduce an intravenous catheter through a region that has partial-thickness burns.
A. True
B. False

_____ 139. What special facility/service might benefit the patient with carbon monoxide poisoning?
A. the burn center
B. trauma center
C. a hospital with thoracic surgery available
D. hyperbaric chamber
E. none of the above

_____ 140. The cyanide antidote kit contains which of the following?
A. amyl nitrate
B. sodium nitrate
C. sodium thiosulfate
D. all of the above
E. none of the above

_____ 141. The paramedic can presume that a high-tension electrical line is not energized when it no longer sparks or gives off a blue glow.
A. True
B. False

_____ 142. Lightning strikes account for approximately what number of deaths per year?
A. 5
B. 25
C. 50
D. 75
E. 100

143. Which chemical burn should be covered with the oil used to hold the agent that caused it?
    A. phenol
    B. dry lime
    C. sodium
    D. riot control agents
    E. organophosphate

144. When chemicals are splashed into the eyes of the patient with contacts, the contacts should be left in place because they will protect the underlying corneas.
    A. True
    B. False

145. If it is necessary to enter a radiation zone to remove a patient, which provider is the best candidate to perform the maneuver?
    A. a young female care provider
    B. a young male care provider
    C. the oldest care provider
    D. the fastest care provider
    E. the heaviest care provider

Chapter 7: Musculoskeletal Trauma

146. What percentage of multi-system trauma patients have musculoskeletal injuries?
    A. 20 percent
    B. 40 percent
    C. 50 percent
    D. 60 percent
    E. 80 percent

147. The bone cell responsible for laying down new bone tissue is the:
    A. osteoblast.
    B. osteoclast.
    C. osteocyte.
    D. osteocrit.
    E. osteophage.

148. The widened end of a long bone is called the:
    A. diaphysis.
    B. epiphysis.
    C. metaphysis.
    D. cancellous bone.
    E. compact bone.

149. The bone tissue making up the central portion of the long bone is called the:
    A. diaphysis.
    B. epiphysis.
    C. metaphysis.
    D. cancellous bone.
    E. compact bone.

150. The penetration through the compact bone that permits blood vessels to enter and exit the shaft of the long bones is the:
    A. periosteum.
    B. peritoneum.
    C. perforating canal.
    D. osteocyte.
    E. epiphysis.

151. The body joints that permit free movement are termed:
    A. synovial joints.
    B. synarthroses.
    C. amphiarthroses.
    D. diarthroses.
    E. A or D

152. The shoulder and hip are examples of which type of joint?
    A. monaxial
    B. biaxial
    C. triaxial
    D. synarthrosis
    E. amphiarthrosis

153. Which of the following is a bone of the forearm?
    A. humerus
    B. radius
    C. olecranon
    D. phalange
    E. carpal

_____ 154. Which of the following is the bump of the elbow?
A. humerus   D. phalange
B. radius   E. carpal
C. olecranon

_____ 155. Which of the following is the major bone of the lower leg?
A. tarsal   D. femur
B. tibia   E. phalange
C. fibula

_____ 156. At what age does the degeneration of bone tissue generally begin?
A. 10   D. 50
B. 20   E. 62
C. 40

_____ 157. Which of the following is not a classification of muscle tissue?
A. cardiac   D. involuntary
B. smooth   E. contractile
C. voluntary

_____ 158. The strong bands of connective tissue securing muscle to bone are the:
A. bursae.   D. cartilage.
B. tendons.   E. meninges.
C. ligaments.

_____ 159. The muscle attachment to the bone that does NOT move when the muscle mass contracts is the:
A. flexor.   D. insertion.
B. extensor.   E. articulation.
C. origin.

_____ 160. The condition which is caused by overstretching of some muscle fibers and which produces pain in the affected muscle group is called:
A. cramp.   D. sprain.
B. fatigue.   E. spasm.
C. strain.

_____ 161. The partial displacement of a bone end from its location within a joint capsule is a:
A. strain.   D. spasm.
B. sprain.   E. subluxation.
C. cramp.

_____ 162. Which of the following fractures is caused by a rotational injury mechanism?
A. hairline   D. comminuted
B. oblique   E. spiral
C. transverse

_____ 163. The greenstick fracture is an incomplete fracture that occasionally must be completely broken to permit proper healing.
A. True
B. False

_____ 164. A common and serious type of fracture occurring in the pediatric patient that may prevent normal bone growth is the:
A. hairline.   D. comminuted.
B. oblique.   E. spiral.
C. epiphyseal.

_____ 165. A chronic, systemic, and progressive deterioration of the connective tissue in the peripheral joints describes:
  A. gout.
  B. rheumatoid arthritis.
  C. osteoarthritis.
  D. bursitis.
  E. tendinitis.

_____ 166. A degenerative disease related to the normal wear and tear of the joint tissue describes:
  A. gout.
  B. rheumatoid arthritis.
  C. osteoarthritis.
  D. bursitis.
  E. tendinitis.

_____ 167. If a fracture of the pelvis or of bilateral femurs is suspected and patient vital signs are stable, the PASG should be:
  A. inflated to pop-off pressure.
  B. inflated until immobilization is achieved.
  C. applied but not inflated until vital signs begin to fall.
  D. withheld and the long spine board and traction splint used instead.
  E. none of the above

_____ 168. Which of the following signs is reflective of a fracture?
  A. distal pulse loss
  B. crepitus
  C. false motion
  D. deformity
  E. all of the above

_____ 169. An elderly patient who has suffered a fracture due to bone degeneration is expected to experience what level of pain when compared to the traumatic fracture experienced by a younger adult patient?
  A. about the same
  B. more pain
  C. less pain
  D. no pain at all
  E. extreme pain

_____ 170. Musculoskeletal injuries associated with sports are generally less severe than trauma-induced injuries and should merit a quick return to competition if possible.
  A. True
  B. False

_____ 171. Only attempt manipulation of a dislocation if a neurovascular deficit is noted.
  A. True
  B. False

_____ 172. In general, most fractures should be left in the position found because the splints of today are very effective in immobilizing a limb in that position.
  A. True
  B. False

_____ 173. Descending in altitude in a helicopter will cause the pressure in the air splint to:
  A. increase.
  B. decrease.
  C. remain the same.
  D. become less uniform.
  E. become more uniform.

_____ 174. The traction splint is designed to splint which musculoskeletal injury?
  A. knee dislocation
  B. hip dislocation
  C. pelvic fracture
  D. femur fracture
  E. all of the above

_____ 175. Align an angulated long bone fracture unless:
  A. pulses are absent distal to the injury.
  B. there is a significant increase in pain.
  C. both sensation and pulses are intact.
  D. sensation is absent distal to the injury.
  E. motor function is absent distal to the injury.

176. If after moving a limb to alignment you notice distal sensation is absent, you should:
  A. splint the limb, as is.
  B. gently move the limb to restore the pulse.
  C. return the limb to the original positioning.
  D. elevate the limb and then splint it.
  E. none of the above

177. Signs that a reduction of a dislocation has been effective include which of the following?
  A. feeling a "pop"
  B. the patient reporting less pain
  C. the joint becoming more mobile
  D. the joint deformity becoming less
  E. all of the above

178. If the reduction is successful and pulses and sensation are intact, splint the limb in the position of function and transport.
  A. True
  B. False

179. The splinting device recommended for a pelvic fracture is the:
  A. traction splint.
  B. PASG.
  C. spine board and padding.
  D. long padded board splints.
  E. air splint.

180. The splinting device recommended for a painful and isolated fracture of the femur associated with a pelvic fracture is the:
  A. traction splint.
  B. PASG.
  C. spine board and padding.
  D. long padded board splints.
  E. air splint.

181. The splinting device recommended for an isolated fracture of the clavicle is the:
  A. traction splint.
  B. PASG.
  C. spine board and padding.
  D. air splint.
  E. sling and swathe.

182. The posterior hip dislocation normally presents with the:
  A. foot turned outward.
  B. foot turned inward.
  C. knee flexed.
  D. knee turned inward.
  E. all except A

183. The ankle is deformed with the foot pointing downward. Which type of ankle dislocation do you suspect?
  A. anterior
  B. posterior
  C. lateral
  D. medial
  E. inferior

184. The patient's arm is internally rotated and the elbow and forearm are held away from the chest. What type of dislocation of the shoulder should you suspect?
  A. anterior
  B. inferior
  C. superior
  D. posterior
  E. lateral

185. The arm is held immobile above the shoulder and chest. What type of dislocation of the shoulder do you suspect?
  A. anterior
  B. inferior
  C. superior
  D. posterior
  E. lateral

186. The elbow dislocation should NOT be reduced in the field.
  A. True
  B. False

_____ 187. Which of the following injuries can be adequately splinted using the full-arm air splint and placing the hand in the position of function?
  A. radial fracture
  B. ulnar fracture
  C. wrist fracture
  D. finger fracture
  E. all of the above

_____ 188. All of the following statements are true about nitrous oxide EXCEPT:
  A. It is non-explosive.
  B. It reduces the perception of pain.
  C. It self-administered.
  D. It remains only in the bloodstream.
  E. It is a controlled substance.

_____ 189. For which of the following will naloxone reverse the drug effects?
  A. meperidine
  B. morphine
  C. nalbuphine
  D. diazepam
  E. A, B, and C

_____ 190. The "C" in the acronym RICE used by athletic trainers stands for:
  A. circulation.
  B. compression.
  C. complexion.
  D. communication.
  E. composure.

Chapter 8: Head, Facial, and Neck Trauma

_____ 191. Which of the following groups is at the lowest risk for head injuries?
  A. females 15 to 24 years of age
  B. males 15 to 24 years of age
  C. young children
  D. the elderly
  E. infants

_____ 192. Which of the following is NOT a bone of the cranium?
  A. frontal bone
  B. nasal bone
  C. parietal bone
  D. sphenoid bone
  E. ethmoid bone

_____ 193. Place the following layers of the meninges as they occur from the skull to the cerebrum.
  A. dura mater, pia mater, arachnoid
  B. dura mater, arachnoid, pia mater
  C. arachnoid, pia mater, dura mater
  D. arachnoid, dura mater, pia mater
  E. pia mater, arachnoid, dura mater

_____ 194. The brain structure that is delicate and covers the convolutions of the cerebrum is the:
  A. pia mater.
  B. falx cerebri.
  C. arachnoid.
  D. dura mater.
  E. tentorium.

_____ 195. The structure that separates the cerebrum from the cerebellum is the:
  A. pia mater.
  B. falx cerebri.
  C. arachnoid.
  D. dura mater.
  E. tentorium.

_____ 196. The cerebrum fine tunes motor control and is responsible for balance and muscle tone.
  A. True
  B. False

_____ 197. Which of the following is a function of the hypothalamus?
  A. control of heart rate
  B. balance
  C. thirst
  D. sleep
  E. speech

_____ 198. Which of the following is a function of the medulla oblongata?
  A. control of respiration
  B. balance
  C. thirst
  D. sleep
  E. none of the above

_____ 199. The brain needs a constant supply of blood to provide oxygen, glucose, and thiamine. Without this supply unconsciousness follows in 10 seconds and death occurs in 4 to 6 minutes.
   A. True
   B. False

_____ 200. Which of the following nerves is responsible for pupillary dilation?
   A. CN I
   B. CN III
   C. CN VIII
   D. CN X
   E. CN XII

_____ 201. Which of the following nerves is responsible for the sense of smell?
   A. CN I
   B. CN III
   C. CN VIII
   D. CN X
   E. CN XII

_____ 202. The upper and immovable jaw bone is the:
   A. maxilla.
   B. mandible.
   C. zygoma.
   D. stapes.
   E. pinna.

_____ 203. The external portion of the ear is the:
   A. maxilla.
   B. mandible.
   C. zygoma.
   D. stapes.
   E. pinna.

_____ 204. The structure responsible for hearing sense is the:
   A. ossicle.
   B. cochlea.
   C. semicircular canals.
   D. sinuses.
   E. vitreous humor.

_____ 205. The muscular tissue surrounding the opening through which light travels to contact the light-sensing tissue in the eye is the:
   A. retina.
   B. aqueous humor.
   C. vitreous humor.
   D. pupil.
   E. iris.

_____ 206. The clear delicate tissue covering the sclera is the:
   A. meninges.
   B. conjunctiva.
   C. cornea.
   D. aqueous humor.
   E. vitreous humor.

_____ 207. Which of the following structures is NOT located within the neck?
   A. the jugular veins
   B. the aorta
   C. the vagus nerve
   D. trachea
   E. esophagus

_____ 208. Scalp wounds may present in a manner that confounds assessment.
   A. True
   B. False

_____ 209. The skull fracture that is related to and often involves some of the numerous natural penetrations (foramina) through the skull is the:
   A. depressed skull fracture.
   B. basilar skull fracture.
   C. linear skull fracture.
   D. comminuted skull fracture.
   E. none of the above

_____ 210. The discoloration found just behind the ear and due to basilar skull fracture is:
   A. retroauricular ecchymosis.
   B. bilateral periorbital ecchymosis.
   C. Cullen's sign.
   D. the halo sign.
   E. none of the above

_____ 211. The injury which causes the brain to be damaged on the side of the impact is called a:
A. coup.
B. subdural hematoma.
C. subluxation.
D. contrecoup.
E. concussion.

_____ 212. Which of the following is considered a diffuse injury?
A. cerebral contusion
B. epidural hematoma
C. subdural hematoma
D. intracerebral hemorrhage
E. none of the above

_____ 213. Bleeding between the dura mater and the interior of the cranium is:
A. cerebral contusion.
B. epidural hematoma.
C. subdural hematoma.
D. intracerebral hemorrhage.
E. none of the above

_____ 214. Which of the following is considered a diffuse brain injury?
A. concussion
B. cerebral contusion
C. epidural hematoma
D. intracerebral hemorrhage
E. subdural hematoma

_____ 215. The brain is one of the most perfusion-sensitive organs of the body.
A. True
B. False

_____ 216. As intracranial hemorrhage begins, it displaces venous blood and then:
A. cerebrospinal fluid.
B. the brainstem.
C. arterial blood.
D. oxygen.
E. the meninges.

_____ 217. In the presence of increased intracranial pressure, the body does which of the following to assure cerebral perfusion?
A. increases cardiac output
B. increases heart rate
C. increases systemic blood pressure
D. dilates peripheral blood vessels
E. all of the above

_____ 218. Low levels of carbon dioxide in the blood will cause which of the following?
A. hyperventilation
B. cerebral artery constriction
C. cerebral artery dilation
D. hypertension
E. none of the above

_____ 219. Herniation of the medulla oblongata through the foramen magnum will cause all of the following EXCEPT:
A. respiratory changes.
B. changes in blood pressure.
C. changes in heart rate.
D. pupillary dilation.
E. increased pulse rate.

_____ 220. Blood loss into the cranium in the infant can contribute significantly to shock and hypovolemia.
A. True
B. False

_____ 221. Increasing intracranial pressure is likely to cause pupillary dilation on the contralateral side from the source of the pressure.
A. True
B. False

_____ 222. According to the Le Fort criteria, a fracture involving the entire facial region below the brow ridge is classified as:
A. Le Fort I.
B. Le Fort II.
C. Le Fort III.
D. Le Fort IV.
E. Le Fort V.

_____ 223. Which of the following mechanisms is likely to injure the tympanum?
A. repeated small arms fire at close range
B. an explosion
C. diving injury
D. objects forced into the ear
E. all of the above

_____ 224. The discoloration of the sclera caused by a bursting blood vessel is called:
A. hyphema.
B. retinal detachment.
C. acute retinal artery occlusion.
D. anterior chamber hematoma.
E. subconjunctival hemorrhage.

_____ 225. The patient complains of a dark curtain over a portion of one eye's field of view after head trauma. You should suspect:
A. hyphema.
B. retinal detachment.
C. acute retinal artery occlusion.
D. anterior chamber hematoma.
E. subconjunctival hemorrhage.

_____ 226. Hyperventilation of the head injury patient is recommended to reduce the chances of hypoxia and hypercarbia.
A. True
B. False

_____ 227. If you do not note the halo sign associated with bleeding from the ear, you can safely rule out cerebrospinal fluid leakage and a basilar skull fracture.
A. True
B. False

_____ 228. A patient complaint of double vision is an example of:
A. diplopia.
B. aniscoria.
C. consensual reactivity.
D. synergism.
E. photophobia.

_____ 229. The Glasgow Coma Scale score for a warm rock would be which of the following?
A. 15
B. 12
C. 10
D. 3
E. 0

_____ 230. The patient with a Glasgow Coma Scale score between 9 and 12 is likely to:
A. have a mild head injury.
B. have a moderate head injury.
C. be in a coma.
D. be brain-dead.
E. none of the above

_____ 231. A patient is very disoriented, uses inappropriate words, opens his eyes on verbal command, and can localize pain. He would be assigned what Glasgow Coma Scale score?
A. 14
B. 12
C. 10
D. 8
E. 6

_____ 232. Vomiting is a serious consequence of head injury that may be due either to swallowing blood or head injury.
A. True
B. False

_____ 233. The patient with a large gaping wound to the neck should be placed in which of the following positions?
A. Trendelenburg
B. with the head of the spine board elevated 30 degrees
C. left lateral recumbent position
D. immobilized completely and rolled to his side
E. none of the above

_____ 234. Digital and nasal endotracheal intubation techniques are recommended for the patient with a suspected spine injury.
A. True
B. False

_____ 235. Repeated or prolonged intubation attempts should be avoided because they may induce dysrhythmias and increase intracranial pressure in the head-injured patient.
A. True
B. False

_____ 236. Which of the following airway techniques is NOT acceptable for the patient with suspected basilar skull fracture?
A. orotracheal intubation
B. directed intubation
C. digital intubation
D. nasotracheal intubation
E. rapid sequence intubation

_____ 237. Which of the following is an acceptable method for confirming endotracheal tube placement in the head injury patient?
A. end-tidal CO_2 detector
B. pulse oximeter
C. the absence of epigastric sounds
D. good and bilaterally equal breath sounds
E. all of the above

_____ 238. In some cases of facial trauma, the airway may be so damaged and distorted that cricothyrotomy is the only way to open the airway.
A. True
B. False

_____ 239. It may be necessary to hold direct pressure on wounds of the neck during all of care and transport to control hemorrhage.
A. True
B. False

_____ 240. In the head injury patient you must keep the blood pressure above:
A. 50 mmHg.
B. 60 mmHg.
C. 90 mmHg.
D. 110 mmHg.
E. 120 mmHg.

_____ 241. Which of the following drugs is the first-line drug in the treatment of head injury?
A. oxygen
B. mannitol
C. furosemide
D. succinylcholine
E. morphine

_____ 242. Which of the following paralytics increases ICP and should be used with caution, if at all, for head injury patients?
A. diazepam
B. mannitol
C. vecuronium
D. succinylcholine
E. midazolam

_____ 243. Midazolam may cause vomiting, nausea, and many of the other signs of head injury.
A. True
B. False

_____ 244. Thiamine is a drug that:
A. causes the liver to release glucagon.
B. helps in the production of insulin.
C. helps process glucose through the Krebs cycle.
D. like insulin, helps glucose cross the cell wall.
E. none of the above

_____ 245. If a large open scalp wound is grossly contaminated, removal of gross contaminants and irrigation are indicated.
  A. True
  B. False

Chapter 9: Spinal Trauma

_____ 246. The portion of the vertebral column you can palpate along the thoracic and lumbar spine is the:
  A. spinous process.
  B. transverse process.
  C. vertebral body.
  D. spinal foramen.
  E. lamina.

_____ 247. Which region of the vertebral column has 7 vertebrae?
  A. cervical
  B. thoracic
  C. lumbar
  D. sacral
  E. coccygeal

_____ 248. Which region of the vertebral column has the largest vertebral bodies?
  A. cervical
  B. thoracic
  C. lumbar
  D. sacral
  E. coccygeal

_____ 249. The region of the spine with the closest tolerance between the spinal cord and the interior of the spinal foramen is the:
  A. cervical spine.
  B. thoracic spine.
  C. lumbar spine.
  D. sacral spine.
  E. coccygeal spine.

_____ 250. The nerve tissue responsible for communicating motor impulses from the brain is(are) the:
  A. white matter.
  B. gray matter.
  C. ascending nerve tracts.
  D. descending nerve tracts.
  E. none of the above

_____ 251. The nerve tissue consisting mostly of nerve cell bodies that makes up the central portion of the spinal cord is(are) the:
  A. white matter.
  B. gray matter.
  C. ascending nerve tracts.
  D. descending nerve tracts.
  E. none of the above

_____ 252. The location to use for assessment of the C-7 nerve root is:
  A. the collar region.
  B. the little finger.
  C. the nipple line.
  D. the umbilicus.
  E. the small toe.

_____ 253. The location to use for assessment of the T-4 nerve root is the:
  A. collar region.
  B. little finger.
  C. nipple line.
  D. umbilicus.
  E. small toe.

_____ 254. Which mechanism of spinal injury is likely to be involved with a dive into shallow water?
  A. extension
  B. flexion
  C. lateral bending
  D. axial loading
  E. distraction

_____ 255. Which mechanism of spinal injury is likely to be involved in a frontal impact auto collision where the driver is restrained by a shoulder strap and lap belt?
  A. extension
  B. flexion
  D. axial loading
  E. both A and B

C. lateral bending

_____ 256. Injury to the connective and skeletal tissue of the spinal column does not mean the spinal cord is injured.
  A. True
  B. False

_____ 257. The most frequently injured location along the spinal column is:
  A. C-1/C-2.
  B. C-7.
  C. T-12/L-1.
  D. L-4.
  E. L-5/S-1.

_____ 258. A spinal cord concussion is not likely to produce residual deficit.
  A. True
  B. False

_____ 259. The signs and symptoms of spinal shock are usually permanent and no recovery is expected.
  A. True
  B. False

_____ 260. Which of the following is a sign associated with neurogenic shock.
  A. priapism
  B. decreased heart rate
  C. decreased peripheral vascular resistance
  D. cool skin above the injury
  E. all of the above

_____ 261. In which type of shock can some recovery of function be expected after the initial injury?
  A. autonomic hyperreflexia syndrome
  B. neurogenic shock
  C. spinal shock
  D. central cord syndrome
  E. both C and D

_____ 262. Which of the following is a mechanism of injury likely to cause spinal injury?
  A. fall from over three times the patient's height
  B. high-speed motor vehicle crash
  C. serious blunt trauma above the shoulders
  D. open wounds directed toward the spine
  E. all of the above

_____ 263. If you are unclear about the mechanism of injury or the potential for spinal injury, always err on the side of caution.
  A. True
  B. False

_____ 264. Digital intubation may be a useful technique in the spinal injury patient because it permits spinal movement without endangering the cord.
  A. True
  B. False

_____ 265. The pulse rate in the patient with high spinal injury is likely to be:
  A. fast.
  B. very fast.
  C. slow.
  D. very slow.
  E. normal.

_____ 266. During your assessment of a patient, you find sensation is lost as you move from the lower extremities all the way up to the level of the umbilicus. This is probably due to an injury at which spinal level?
  A. C-3
  B. C-7
  C. T-4
  D. T-10
  E. S-1

_____ 267. Which of the following is indicative of spinal injury?
 A. increased heart rate
 B. increasing blood pressure
 C. rapid, deep breathing
 D. abnormal body temperature, often related to environmental temperatures
 E. none of the above

_____ 268. The ideal positioning for the spine includes the patient's nose in line with which of the following?
 A. clavicle
 B. shoulders
 C. navel
 D. wrists
 E. all of the above

_____ 269. The most ideal position for the infant's head during spinal immobilization is:
 A. 2 to 3 inches above the spine board.
 B. level with the spine board.
 C. with padding under the shoulders on the spine board.
 D. with the head slightly extended and level with the spine board.
 E. none of the above

_____ 270. Which of the criteria below indicates that a helmet should be removed from a patient?
 A. The head is not immobilized within the helmet.
 B. The helmet prevents airway maintenance.
 C. You cannot secure the helmet firmly to the long spine board.
 D. You anticipate breathing problems.
 E. any of the above

_____ 271. Proper helmet removal requires a minimum of how many care providers?
 A. 2
 B. 3
 C. 4
 D. 5
 E. no less than 6

_____ 272. Prior to initiating a log roll, it is preferable to place a bulky blanket between the legs.
 A. True
 B. False

_____ 273. The log roll for the patient with spinal injuries requires a minimum of how many care providers?
 A. 2
 B. 3
 C. 4
 D. 5
 E. no less than 6

_____ 274. To immobilize the patient's head to the long spine board, you should use a:
 A. cervical collar.
 B. vest-type immobilization device.
 C. cervical immobilization device.
 D. vacuum splint.
 E. any of the above

_____ 275. You immobilize the patient's head to the long spine board before you secure his body to it.
 A. True
 B. False

Chapter 10: Thoracic Trauma

_____ 276. In vehicular accidents, chest trauma accounts for:
 A. the greatest cause of mortality.
 B. 25 percent of the mortality.
 C. the third greatest cause of mortality.
 D. a minor incidence of mortality.
 E. none of the above

_____ 277. Which of the following is located within the thorax?
  A. the vagus nerve   D. the bronchi
  B. the aortic arch   E. all of the above
  C. the superior vena cava

_____ 278. Which muscle group lifts the sternum and, with it, the thoracic cage to assist with respiration?
  A. the intercostals   D. the scalenes
  B. the diaphragm   E. the rectus abdominis
  C. the sternocleidomastoids

_____ 279. At the beginning of and during most of inhalation the pressure within the thorax is:
  A. less than that of the environment.
  B. more than that of the environment.
  C. equal to the that of the environment.
  D. first lower than and then higher than that of the environment.
  E. first higher than and then lower than that of the environment.

_____ 280. The location where the pulmonary arteries and the mainstem bronchus enter the lung is the:
  A. pleura.   D. cardiac notch.
  B. pulmonary hilum.   E. carina.
  C. ligamentum arteriosum.

_____ 281. The oxygen in the air we exhale is about:
  A. 79 percent.   D. 4 percent.
  B. 21 percent.   E. 0.04 percent.
  C. 16 percent.

_____ 282. The carbon dioxide content of the air we breathe in is about:
  A. 79 percent.   D. 4 percent.
  B. 21 percent.   E. 0.04 percent.
  C. 16 percent.

_____ 283. The maximum volume of air forcefully exhaled after an maximum inhalation is the:
  A. residual volume.   D. vital capacity.
  B. dead space volume.   E. inspiratory capacity.
  C. tidal volume.

_____ 284. The volume of air left in the lungs after a maximal exhalation is the:
  A. residual volume.   D. vital capacity.
  B. dead space volume.   E. inspiratory capacity.
  C. tidal volume.

_____ 285. Which of the following monitor(s) oxygen levels to stimulate respiration?
  A. chemoreceptors in the carotid bodies
  B. chemoreceptors in the medulla oblongata
  C. the apneustic center
  D. chemoreceptors in the aortic bodies
  E. both A and D

_____ 286. The more internal the myocardium, the more susceptible it is to ischemia.
  A. True
  B. False

_____ 287. The sac surrounding the heart is called the:
  A. myocardium.   D. parietal cardiac sheath.
  B. endocardium.   E. epicardium arteriosum.
  C. pericardium.

_____ 288. The muscular layer of the heart is the:
  A. fibrous pericardium.   D. endocardium.
  B. epicardium.   E. myocardium.
  C. pericardium.

_____ 289. The structure that connects the aorta to the pulmonary artery and holds it in position within the thorax is the:
  A. pleura.   D. epicardium pocket.
  B. pulmonary hilum.   E. vena cava.
  C. ligamentum arteriosum.

_____ 290. Which of the following is NOT likely to be associated with blunt trauma?
  A. flail chest
  B. pneumothorax (paper bag syndrome)
  C. open pneumothorax
  D. aortic aneurysm
  E. myocardial contusion

_____ 291. Which of the following is NOT likely to be associated with penetrating trauma?
  A. pericardial tamponade   D. aortic aneurysm
  B. tracheal disruption   E. comminuted rib fracture
  C. open pneumothorax

_____ 292. Which pairs of ribs most frequently transmit kinetic energy and trauma to the tissues beneath them without fracturing?
  A. ribs 1 and 2   D. ribs 9 through 12
  B. ribs 3 and 4   E. both A and B
  C. ribs 4 through 8

_____ 293. Which of the following patients is most likely to experience rib fracture with the least force of trauma?
  A. the infant patient   D. the elderly patient
  B. the adult male patient   E. the child patient
  C. the adult female patient

_____ 294. A flail segment moves in opposition to the chest wall during paradoxical movement.
  A. True
  B. False

_____ 295. As time passes, the continuing injury and muscle fatigue will permit the amount of paradoxical movement to increase with a flail chest injury.
  A. True
  B. False

_____ 296. Which patient is most likely to display tracheal deviation early in the course of a tension pneumothorax?
  A. the pediatric patient   D. the pregnant patient
  B. the young adult patient   E. the elderly patient
  C. the older adult patient

_____ 297. Each side of the thorax can hold up to half the patient's total blood supply. Hence, hemothorax is often a more of a hypovolemic problem with limited respiratory signs and symptoms.
  A. True
  B. False

_____ 298. Pulmonary contusion may result from:
  A. a bullet's passage.
  B. traumatic chest compression.
  C. the over-pressure wave of a strong explosion.
  D. high-velocity bullet striking body armor.
  E. all of the above

_____ 299. Which of the following is NOT associated with a pulmonary contusion?
  A. atelectasis
  B. increased respiratory effort
  C. increased rate of carbon dioxide diffusion
  D. microhemorrhage into the alveolar tissue
  E. decreased rate of oxygen diffusion

_____ 300. Myocardial contusion may result in all of the following EXCEPT:
  A. ectopic beats.
  B. heart blocks.
  C. hemoperitoneum.
  D. subcutaneous emphysema.
  E. decreased ventricular compliance.

_____ 301. Which of the following is the most frequent mechanism of injury causing pericardial tamponade?
  A. blunt anterior chest trauma
  B. penetrating chest trauma
  C. the blast pressure wave
  D. traumatic asphyxia
  E. lateral impact auto crash

_____ 302. Which of the following is a sign of pericardial tamponade?
  A. cyanosis of the upper extremities and head
  B. decreased JVD during inspiration
  C. electrical alternans
  D. pulseless electrical activity
  E. all of the above

_____ 303. Jugular vein distention, distant heart tones, and hypotension are collectively known as:
  A. Beck's triad.
  B. pulsus paradoxus.
  C. Cushing's reflex.
  D. Kussmaul's sign.
  E. electrical alternans.

_____ 304. Which of the following is the most frequent mechanism of injury causing traumatic aortic aneurysm?
  A. blunt anterior chest trauma
  B. penetrating chest trauma
  C. the blast pressure wave
  D. traumatic asphyxia
  E. lateral impact auto crash

_____ 305. Which of the following is a point of fixation for the aorta in the thorax?
  A. the diaphragm
  B. the aortic annulus
  C. the aortic isthmus
  D. all of the above
  E. none of the above

_____ 306. The left side is the site of most diaphragmatic ruptures because most assailants are right-handed.
  A. True
  B. False

_____ 307. Which of the following may cause the abdomen to appear hollow?
  A. traumatic asphyxia
  B. tension pneumothorax
  C. aortic aneurysm
  D. diaphragmatic rupture
  E. none of the above

_____ 308. Tracheobronchial disruption is likely to occur at what location?
  A. more than 2.5 cm below the carina
  B. more than 2.5 cm above the carina
  C. within 2.5 cm of the carina
  D. at the bronchial bifurcation
  E. along the right mainstem bronchus

_____ 309. The greatest problems associated with traumatic asphyxia are related to the:
  A. bellows system.
  B. airway.
  C. heart.
  D. vasculature.
  E. lung tissue.

310. While assessing a supine patient, the jugular veins are found distended. This finding alone suggests:
A. a normal patient.
B. pericardial tamponade.
C. tension pneumothorax.
D. traumatic asphyxia.
E. B, C, and D

311. A dull percussion noted in the lower lobe of a lung is suggestive of:
A. pneumothorax.
B. tension pneumothorax.
C. hemothorax.
D. pulmonary contusion.
E. both A and B

312. Overdrive ventilation (bag-valve masking) of the patient with pulmonary contusions and developing edema may help push fluids back into the lung tissues.
A. True
B. False

313. You have covered the open pneumothorax in a thoracic injury patient. You then notice that dyspnea is increasing and breath sounds on the injured side are becoming diminished. Which action would you take?
A. Insert a needle in the 2nd intercostal space.
B. Remove the dressing.
C. Provide overdrive ventilation.
D. Consider nitrous oxide administration.
E. all of the above

314. Which location is recommended for prehospital pleural decompression?
A. 2nd intercostal space, midclavicular line
B. 5th intercostal space, midclavicular line
C. 5th intercostal space, midaxillary line
D. A and B
E. A and C

315. Which of the following drugs would be considered for the patient who has experienced traumatic asphyxia for more than 20 minutes?
A. decadron
B. sodium bicarbonate
C. morphine sulfate
D. demerol
E. dopamine

Chapter 11: Abdominal Trauma

316. Which of the following abdominal organs is found in the left lower quadrant?
A. the spleen
B. the gallbladder
C. the appendix
D. sigmoid colon
E. none of the above

317. Which of the following abdominal organs is found in the right upper quadrant?
A. the spleen
B. the gallbladder
C. the appendix
D. sigmoid colon
E. none of the above

318. Which of the following abdominal organs is found in of all the abdominal quadrants?
A. the spleen
B. the gallbladder
C. the appendix
D. the sigmoid colon
E. the small bowel

319. The organ storing a digestive juice created by the liver is the:
A. spleen.
B. small bowel.
C. pancreas.
D. gallbladder.
E. liver.

_____ 320. The organ where bile and pancreatic juices are mixed with the digesting food is the:
  A. spleen.   D. gallbladder.
  B. small bowel.   E. liver.
  C. stomach.

_____ 321. The urinary bladder may contain as little as 10 mL of fluid or as much as 500 mL of fluid.
  A. True
  B. False

_____ 322. The ovary releases a fertilized egg every 28 days.
  A. True
  B. False

_____ 323. The location where eggs are most commonly fertilized is the:
  A. vagina.   D. ovary.
  B. uterus.   E. cervix.
  C. fallopian tube.

_____ 324. Pregnancy causes what change in the maternal blood volume?
  A. a 10 percent decrease   D. a 45 percent increase
  B. a 25 percent decrease   E. a 65 percent increase
  C. a 25 percent increase

_____ 325. The connective tissue suspending the bowel from the posterior abdominal wall is the:
  A. perineum.   D. retroperitoneum.
  B. mesentery.   E. ileum.
  C. peritoneum.

_____ 326. Penetrating trauma may cause which of the following injuries?
  A. spillage of the contents of hollow organs
  B. hemorrhage from solid organs
  C. damage to organs
  D. eventual irritation of the abdominal lining
  E. all of the above

_____ 327. Blunt mechanisms cause injuries to the spleen about what percentage of the time?
  A. 40 percent   D. 10 percent
  B. 30 percent   E. 5 percent
  C. 20 percent

_____ 328. Penetrating mechanisms injure the small bowel about what percentage of the time?
  A. 40 percent   D. 10 percent
  B. 25 percent   E. 5 percent
  C. 20 percent

_____ 329. Which of the following organs is most frequently damaged during penetrating abdominal trauma?
  A. the small bowel   D. the kidneys
  B. the liver   E. the pancreas
  C. the spleen

_____ 330. Penetration of the abdominal wall where the abdominal contents protrude is called:
  A. peritonitis.   D. peristalsis.
  B. chyme.   E. emulsification.
  C. evisceration.

_____ 331. Most abdominal vascular injuries are associated with blunt trauma.
  A. True
  B. False

_____ 332. Which of the following is NOT true regarding abdominal vascular injury and hemorrhage?
A. Intra-abdominal pressure associated with those injuries does not restrict hemorrhage.
B. Blood-induced irritation of the abdominal lining occurs quickly.
C. Hemorrhage can accumulate without any swelling becoming apparent.
D. Blood in the abdomen may trigger a vagal response, slowing the heart.
E. The abdomen has many large arterial and venous structures.

_____ 333. An injury associated with the release of either blood or bowel contents into the abdominal cavity will result in a rapidly developing presentation of severe discomfort and pain.
A. True
B. False

_____ 334. Gastric or duodenal contents released into the abdominal space will irritate the peritoneum faster than bacteria will.
A. True
B. False

_____ 335. The late term female is at decreased risk for vomiting and aspiration.
A. True
B. False

_____ 336. Supine positioning of the mother may cause hypotension due to:
A. decreased intra-abdominal pressure.
B. compression of the inferior vena cava.
C. increased intra-abdominal pressure.
D. increased circulation to the uterus.
E. none of the above

_____ 337. The signs of abdominal trauma may become less specific due to the progression of peritonitis.
A. True
B. False

_____ 338. Penetrating trauma just under the right thoracic border is likely to injure the:
A. liver.   D. bladder.
B. spleen.   E. left kidney.
C. bowel.

_____ 339. The major reason auscultation of bowel and other abdominal sounds is not recommended in the field is because:
A. the sounds are not clear.
B. the sounds do not rule out injury.
C. the lack of sounds does not confirm injury.
D. it takes too long to adequately assess bowel sounds.
E. B, C, and D

_____ 340. The abdominal evisceration covered with a moist dressing should then be covered with a(n):
A. dry, adherent dressing and wrapped firmly.
B. dry, nonadherent dressing and wrapped loosely.
C. damp, nonadherent dressing wrapped loosely.
D. occlusive dressing and wrapped loosely.
E. damp, nonadherent dressing wrapped firmly.

Chapter 12: Shock Trauma Resuscitation

_____ 341. In the United States, trauma is the:
   A. leading cause of death.
   B. second-leading cause of death.
   C. third-leading cause of death.
   D. fourth-leading cause of death.
   E. fifth-leading cause of death.

_____ 342. The annual death toll from trauma is around:
   A. 38,000.
   B. 44,000.
   C. 85,000.
   D. 150,000.
   E. 200,000.

_____ 343. An EMS home inspection might examine for:
   A. knowledge of children's auto seat.
   B. helmet usage.
   C. outlet covers in children's spaces.
   D. knowledge of how to access EMS.
   E. all of the above

_____ 344. The anticipation of specific injuries gained from the analysis of the mechanism of injury is the:
   A. factor of severity.
   B. index of suspicion.
   C. revised trauma score.
   D. trauma score.
   E. none of the above

_____ 345. If the hazardous materials team is not yet on scene and the patient is found to have suffered serious injuries, you would be responsible for removing him from the site and to an area free of contamination.
   A. True
   B. False

_____ 346. The risk of contamination and resultant disease from contact with body substances is greater for your patient than for you.
   A. True
   B. False

_____ 347. A patient with airway trauma and serious airway bleeding suggests what items of personal protection for the paramedic?
   A. gloves
   B. gloves and goggles
   C. gloves and gown
   D. gloves and mask
   E. gloves, goggles, mask, and gown

_____ 348. Air medical service should be summoned for any serious trauma scene more than which distance/time from the trauma center?
   A. 20 to 30 minutes
   B. 4 miles
   C. 10 miles
   D. 2 miles
   E. 30 to 40 minutes

_____ 349. Which of the following is NOT an element of the initial assessment?
   A. spinal precautions
   B. a general patient impression
   C. SAMPLE history
   D. airway maintenance
   E. serious hemorrhage control

_____ 350. The "P" of the AVPU mnemonic stands for:
   A. positional sense
   B. posturing
   C. pain
   D. purposeful
   E. proprioception

_____ 351. Which of the following levels of orientation correctly represents the order in which they are lost?
   A. persons, time, place
   B. time, persons, place
   C. place, persons, time
   D. time, place, persons
   E. persons, place, time

_____ 352. The movement by the patient to a position of muscular extension with the elbows extending is termed:
  A. purposeful.
  B. purposeless.
  C. decorticate posturing.
  D. decerebrate posturing.
  E. painful.

_____ 353. If you are required to ventilate a patient, what volume of air would you use for breaths?
  A. 500 mL
  B. 600 mL
  C. 800 to 1,000 mL
  D. 1,000 to 1,200 mL
  E. 1,200 to 1,500 mL

_____ 354. Capillary refill is no longer of value in the assessment of the adult patient.
  A. True
  B. False

_____ 355. Which of the following will affect the rate of capillary refill in the adult patient?
  A. smoking
  B. low ambient temperatures
  C. pre-existing disease
  D. medications
  E. all of the above

_____ 356. A patient's perception of pain levels is subjective, and different people have different pain tolerances.
  A. True
  B. False

_____ 357. Percussion of the chest may yield a dull response with:
  A. blood accumulation.
  B. fluid accumulation.
  C. air.
  D. air under pressure.
  E. both A and B

_____ 358. Components of the detailed physical exam are used rarely in prehospital trauma care.
  A. True
  B. False

_____ 359. When one eye is exposed to a strong light, the opposite pupil should:
  A. remain as it is.
  B. dilate briskly.
  C. dilate slowly.
  D. constrict briskly.
  E. constrict slowly.

_____ 360. It is important to identify use of which of the following when obtaining a history of the trauma patient?
  A. aspirin
  B. anticoagulants
  C. beta blockers
  D. antibiotics
  E. all of the above

_____ 361. Which of the following is NOT an indication of shock compensation?
  A. shallow respirations
  B. an increasing pulse rate
  C. a decreasing level of consciousness
  D. an increasing pulse strength
  E. cool and clammy skin

_____ 362. A trauma patient is breathing at 24 times per minute, has normal respiratory expansion, a blood pressure of 80 systolic, delayed capillary refill of 4 seconds, and a Glasgow Coma Scale score of 12. What should you report to medical direction as the revised trauma score?
  A. 7
  B. 9
  C. 10
  D. 11
  E. 15

_____ 363. The ongoing assessment should be preformed every 5 minutes on the seriously injured trauma patient.
  A. True
  B. False

_____ 364. Which of the following is a term that refers to lower than normal blood pressure?
  A. hypovolemia
  B. hypoperfusion
  C. hypotension
  D. anemia
  E. none of the above

_____ 365. Which of the following is a word that means "shock"?
  A. hypovolemia
  B. hypoperfusion
  C. hypotension
  D. anemia
  E. hypertension

_____ 366. Hypothermia is a common complication of shock.
  A. True
  B. False

_____ 367. Which of the following is NOT true regarding pediatric patients when compared to adults?
  A. Their limbs are shorter and less able to protect the trunk.
  B. Their skeletons are better able to protect internal organs.
  C. Their airways are smaller.
  D. They compensate for blood loss better.
  E. Their skeletal components are more flexible.

_____ 368. Which of the following is NOT true regarding the changes in vital signs with advancing age?
  A. The blood pressure increases.
  B. The pulse rate decreases.
  C. The respirations slow.
  D. The body temperature rises.
  E. The respiratory volume increases.

_____ 369. The oral airway should be inserted by rotating it 180 degrees during insertion for the pediatric patient.
  A. True
  B. False

_____ 370. The maximum recommended fluid administration volume for a pediatric trauma patient is:
  A. 1,000 mL.
  B. 2,000 mL.
  C. 20 mL/kg.
  D. 60 mL/kg.
  E. 80 mL/kg.

_____ 371. Which of the following is generally NOT true regarding elderly patients?
  A. Their bones are more brittle.
  B. Their renal function is decreased.
  C. Their brain mass and volume are decreased.
  D. Their pain perception is heightened.
  E. Their cardiac strike volume is decreased.

_____ 372. Key elements of the verbal patient care report include all of the following EXCEPT:
  A. mechanism of injury.
  B. interventions.
  C. results of assessment.
  D. names of EMS personnel.
  E. results of interventions.

_____ 373. The landing zone for a large-sized helicopter should be at least:
  A. 25 by 25 feet.
  B. 40 by 40 feet.
  C. 60 by 60 feet.
  D. 75 by 75 feet.
  E. 120 by 120 feet.

_____ 374. Increasing altitude in a helicopter is likely to cause:
   A. the pressure in an endotracheal cuff to decrease.
   B. the pressure of a tension pneumothorax to decrease.
   C. the pressure in the PASG to decrease.
   D. oxygen saturation to decrease.
   E. the severity of asthma to decrease.

_____ 375. Which of the following is essential in preparing the trauma patient for air medical flight?
   A. assuring a secure airway
   B. completely immobilizing the patient to a long spine board
   C. assuring maximal oxygenation
   D. establishing two good IV lines
   E. all of the above

WORKBOOK ANSWER KEY

Note: Throughout Answer Key, textbook page references are shown in italic.

CHAPTER 1: Trauma and Trauma Systems

CONTENT SELF-EVALUATION

MULTIPLE CHOICE

1. C *p. 5*	6. D *p. 6*	11. A *p. 11*
2. A *p. 5*	7. B *p. 7*	12. A *p. 11*
3. A *p. 5*	8. D *p. 7*	13. E *p. 13*
4. A *p. 6*	9. E *p. 8*	14. C *p. 13*
5. C *p. 6*	10. B *p. 10*	15. A *p. 14*

CHAPTER 2: Blunt Trauma

CONTENT SELF-EVALUATION

MULTIPLE CHOICE

1. A *p. 19*	15. C *p. 28*	29. A *p. 41*
2. B *p. 19*	16. B *p. 28*	30. E *p. 42*
3. B *p. 19*	17. C *p. 29*	31. D *p. 44*
4. D *p. 20*	18. A *p. 32*	32. B *p. 44*
5. C *p. 20*	19. E *p. 32*	33. C *p. 45*
6. E *p. 20*	20. A *p. 34*	34. A *p. 45*
7. B *p. 21*	21. E *p. 35*	35. C *p. 46*
8. E *p. 22*	22. E *p. 36*	36. A *p. 46*
9. E *p. 23*	23. B *p. 36*	37. D *p. 47*
10. D *p. 24*	24. D *p. 37*	38. B *p. 48*
11. A *p. 26*	25. A *p. 37*	39. A *p. 50*
12. B *p. 26*	26. E *p. 38*	40. E *p. 51*
13. C *p. 27*	27. C *p. 39*	
14. B *p. 28*	28. A *p. 40*	

SPECIAL PROJECT: Injury Mechanism Analysis

A. Mechanism of injury: sports injury, blunt trauma. Anticipated injuries: head (but well-protected); neck/spine, skeletal—fractures and/or dislocations; muscular—sprains, strains.

B. Mechanism of injury: frontal impact auto crash. Anticipated injuries: head injury; cervical spine injury; chest injury; abdominal injury; foot, leg, and thigh injuries.

C. Mechanism of injury: explosion, pressure wave, projectiles, structural collapse. Anticipated injuries: pressure wave—lung, bowel, ear injuries; penetrating trauma from projectiles; burns; inhalation injuries; blunt trauma; crush injuries.

CHAPTER 3: Penetrating Trauma

CONTENT SELF-EVALUATION

MULTIPLE CHOICE

1. B *p. 56*	7. A *p. 60*	13. E *p. 66*
2. C *p. 57*	8. B *p. 60*	14. D *p. 66*
3. A *p. 57*	9. E *p. 62*	15. C *p. 67*
4. C *p. 58*	10. A *p. 63*	16. B *p. 68*
5. B *p. 59*	11. A *p. 65*	17. A *p. 69*
6. E *p. 59*	12. C *p. 66*	18. A *p. 69*

19. A *p. 70*	22. B *p. 71*	24. D *p. 73*
20. D *p. 70*	23. E *p. 72*	25. C *p. 74*
21. C *p. 71*		

SPECIAL PROJECT: Label the Diagram

A. Zone of injury
B. Permanent cavity
C. Pressure wave
D. Temporary cavity
E. Direct injury

CHAPTER 4: Hemorrhage and Shock

CONTENT SELF-EVALUATION

MULTIPLE CHOICE

1. C *p. 79*	21. C *p. 90*	41. D *p. 106*
2. E *p. 79*	22. E *p. 91*	42. C *p. 106*
3. B *p. 80*	23. D *p. 91*	43. B *p. 108*
4. B *p. 80*	24. A *p. 91*	44. B *p. 108*
5. C *p. 81*	25. A *p. 92*	45. A *p. 108*
6. C *p. 81*	26. A *p. 93*	46. C *p. 109*
7. B *p. 81*	27. C *p. 94*	47. B *p. 110*
8. D *p. 81*	28. B *p. 95*	48. C *p. 110*
9. C *p. 82*	29. E *p. 95*	49. B *p. 110*
10. D *p. 83*	30. E *p. 96*	50. C *p. 111*
11. B *p. 83*	31. E *p. 97*	51. E *p. 112*
12. A *p. 84*	32. D *p. 97*	52. D *p. 112*
13. D *p. 84*	33. B *p. 98*	53. A *p. 113*
14. D *p. 84*	34. A *p. 100*	54. B *p. 114*
15. B *p. 84*	35. D *p. 100*	55. E *p. 115*
16. E *p. 85*	36. E *p. 101*	56. C *p. 115*
17. A *p. 85*	37. A *p. 102*	57. E *p. 116*
18. B *p. 88*	38. B *p. 104*	58. B *p. 116*
19. A *p. 89*	39. E *p. 104*	59. E *p. 117*
20. B *p. 90*	40. D *p. 105*	60. A *p. 118*

SPECIAL PROJECT: Scenario-Based Problem Solving

1. liver, kidney, large bowel, small bowel, pancreas, diaphragm

2. The agitation could be related to the nature of his injury and the attack, or he could be experiencing minor cerebral hypoxia due to hypovolemia which will also cause some agitation.

3. An increase in peripheral vascular resistance may be the body's compensation for a decreased cardiac output due to hypovolemia.

4. The increased diastolic pressure (in the absence of an increase in the systolic blood pressure) decreases the pulse pressure. The pulse pressure is the strength of the pulse.

5. The skin becomes cool and clammy as the arterioles serving it constrict to shunt blood to more immediately critical organs like the heart, brain, kidneys, and (to fight or flee) the skeletal muscles.

Drip Math Worksheet 1

1. R = 120 gtts/min
   V = ?
   T = 35 min
   D = 10 gtts/mL

   V = R × T = 120 gtts/min × 35 min

   $$V = \frac{120 \text{ gtts} \times 35 \text{ min}}{\text{min}} = 4200 \text{ gtts}$$

   $$V = \frac{4200 \text{ gtts/D}}{10 \text{ gtts}} = 4200 \text{ gtts} \times \text{mL}$$ **= 420 mL**

2. R = 45 gtts/min
   D = 60 gtts/mL
   D′ = 45 gtts/mL

   R(mL) = R(min)/D = 45 gtts/min/60 gtts/mL

   $$R(mL) = \frac{45 \text{ gtts} \times \text{mL}}{60 \text{ gtts} \times \text{min}} = \frac{45 \text{ mL}}{60 \text{ min}} = 0.75 \text{ mL/min}$$

   R(min) = R(mL) × D′ = 0.75 mL/min × 45 gtts/mL

   $$R(min) = \frac{0.75 \text{ mL} \times 45 \text{ gtts}}{\text{mL} \times \text{min}} = 33.75 \text{ gtts/min}$$

   R(sec) = 33.75 gtts/60 sec   **= 0.56 gtts/sec**

3. R = ?
   V = 100 mL
   T = 115 min
   D = 60 gtts/mL

   R = V/T = 100 mL/115 min = 0.87 mL/min

   R(min) = R(mL) × D = 0.87 mL/min × 60 gtts/min

   $$R(min) = \frac{0.87 \text{ mL} \times 60 \text{ gtts}}{\text{min} \times \text{mL}}$$ **= 52 gtts/min**

4. R = ?
   V = 45 > 100 mL
   T = 60 min
   D = 60 − 45 − 10 gtts/mL
   R(min) = R(mL) × D

   R = V/T = 45 mL/60 min = 0.75 mL/min

   R′ = V/T = 100 mL/60 min = 1.67 mL/min

   $$R(60) = \frac{0.75 \text{ mL/min} \times 60 \text{ gtts/mL}}{\text{min} \times \text{mL}} = 0.75 \text{ mL} \times 60 \text{ gtts}$$ **= 45 gtts/min**

   $$R'(60) = \frac{1.67 \text{ mL/min} \times 60 \text{ gtts/mL}}{\text{min} \times \text{mL}} = 1.67 \text{ mL} \times 60 \text{ gtts}$$ **= 100 gtts/mL**

   $$R(45) = \frac{0.75 \text{ mL/min} \times 45 \text{ gtts/mL}}{\text{min} \times \text{mL}} = 0.75 \text{ mL} \times 45 \text{ gtts}$$ **= 33.75 gtts/min**

   $$R'(45) = \frac{1.67 \text{ mL/min} \times 45 \text{ gtts/mL}}{\text{min} \times \text{mL}} = 1.67 \text{ mL} \times 45 \text{ gtts}$$ **= 75 gtts/mL**

   $$R(10) = \frac{0.75 \text{ mL/min} \times 10 \text{ gtts/mL}}{\text{min} \times \text{mL}} = 0.75 \text{ mL} \times 10 \text{ gtts}$$ **= 7.5 gtts/min**

   $$R'(10) = \frac{1.67 \text{ mL/min} \times 10 \text{ gtts/mL}}{\text{min} \times \text{mL}} = 1.67 \text{ mL} \times 10 \text{ gtts}$$ **= 16.7 gtts/mL**

5. R = ?
   V = 150 mL
   T = 65 min

   $$R = V/T = 150 \text{ mL/65 min} = \frac{150 \text{ mL}}{65 \text{ min}}$$ **= 2.3 mL/min**

CHAPTER 5: Soft-Tissue Trauma

CONTENT SELF-EVALUATION
MULTIPLE CHOICE

1.	B	p. 126	20.	C	p. 139	39.	A	p. 154
2.	A	p. 127	21.	B	p. 139	40.	E	p. 156
3.	E	p. 127	22.	A	p. 139	41.	C	p. 157
4.	D	p. 128	23.	E	p. 140	42.	B	p. 157
5.	A	p. 128	24.	C	p. 140	43.	C	p. 159
6.	B	p. 129	25.	E	p. 141	44.	D	p. 159
7.	B	p. 129	26.	A	p. 141	45.	A	p. 160
8.	B	p. 130	27.	E	p. 142	46.	C	p. 161
9.	E	p. 130	28.	E	p. 142	47.	B	p. 161
10.	B	p. 131	29.	A	p. 143	48.	E	p. 162
11.	C	p. 131	30.	A	p. 143	49.	E	p. 163
12.	D	p. 132	31.	A	p. 145	50.	D	p. 164
13.	E	p. 132	32.	C	p. 145	51.	E	p. 164
14.	B	p. 132	33.	E	p. 145	52.	B	p. 165
15.	A	p. 134	34.	D	p. 147	53.	A	p. 165
16.	D	p. 136	35.	A	p. 148	54.	E	p. 166
17.	B	p. 136	36.	A	p. 149	55.	C	p. 166
18.	B	p. 137	37.	E	p. 150			
19.	B	p. 138	38.	B	p. 154			

CHAPTER 6: Burns

CONTENT SELF-EVALUATION
MULTIPLE CHOICE

1.	A	p. 172	21.	B	p. 186	41.	B	p. 196
2.	D	p. 173	22.	C	p. 186	42.	B	p. 197
3.	C	p. 173	23.	B	p. 186	43.	B	p. 197
4.	D	p. 175	24.	C	p. 186	44.	A	p. 197
5.	A	p. 175	25.	D	p. 186	45.	B	p. 198
6.	D	p. 176	26.	E	p. 186	46.	B	p. 198
7.	B	p. 177	27.	E	p. 187	47.	B	p. 198
8.	A	p. 176	28.	E	p. 189	48.	A	p. 199
9.	C	p. 178	29.	B	p. 191	49.	E	p. 200
10.	E	p. 179	30.	A	p. 192	50.	D	p. 200
11.	A	p. 179	31.	A	p. 192	51.	B	p. 200
12.	B	p. 179	32.	B	p. 192	52.	D	p. 202
13.	C	p. 182	33.	B	p. 192	53.	E	p. 202
14.	A	p. 182	34.	E	p. 193	54.	C	p. 202
15.	E	p. 182	35.	A	p. 195	55.	B	p. 202
16.	D	p. 183	36.	D	p. 195	56.	D	p. 203
17.	B	p. 183	37.	D	p. 195	57.	A	p. 203
18.	E	p. 183	38.	D	p. 195	58.	A	p. 204
19.	C	p. 184	39.	A	p. 196	59.	E	p. 204
20.	D	p. 185	40.	A	p. 196	60.	B	p. 204

SPECIAL PROJECT: Drip Math Worksheet 2

1. R = ?
   T = 2 hour (120 min)
   V = 250 mL

$$\text{Rate} = \frac{\text{Volume}}{\text{Time}} = \frac{250 \text{ mL}}{120 \text{ min}} = \frac{2.08 \text{ mL}}{\text{min}} = 2.08 \text{ mL/min}$$

   A. D = 10 gtts/mL

$$R = V \times D = \frac{2.08 \text{ mL} \times 10 \text{ gtts}}{\text{min} \times \text{mL}} = \frac{20.8 \text{ gtts}}{\text{min}} = 20.8 \text{ gtts/min}$$

   B. D = 15 gtts/mL

$$R = V \times D = \frac{2.08 \text{ mL} \times 15 \text{ gtts}}{\text{min} \times \text{mL}} = \frac{31.2 \text{ gtts}}{\text{min}} = 31.2 \text{ gtts/min}$$

   C. D = 60 gtts/mL

$$R = V \times D = \frac{2.08 \text{ mL} \times 60 \text{ gtts}}{\text{min} \times \text{mL}} = \frac{144 \text{ gtts}}{\text{min}} = 144 \text{ gtts/min}$$

2. R = 30 gtts/min
   T = ?
   D = 60 gtts/mL

$$R = R/D = \frac{30 \text{ gtts} \times \text{mL}}{60 \text{ gtts} \times \text{min}} = \frac{0.5 \text{ mL}}{\text{min}} = 0.5 \text{ mL/min}$$

   A. V = 200

$$T = \frac{V}{R} = \frac{200 \text{ mL} \times \text{min}}{0.5 \text{ mL}} = 400 \text{ min} \quad \frac{400 \text{ min} \times \text{hr}}{60 \text{ min}} = 6.67 \text{ hrs (6 hrs, 40 min)}$$

   B. V = 350

$$T = \frac{V}{R} = \frac{350 \text{ mL} \times \text{min}}{0.5 \text{ mL}} = 700 \text{ min} \quad \frac{700 \text{ min} \times \text{hr}}{60 \text{ min}} = 11.67 \text{ hrs (11 hrs, 40 min)}$$

3. R = 1 gtts/sec = 60 gtts/min
   T = 15 min
   V = ?
   D = 15 gtts/mL

$$R = \frac{60 \text{ gtts} \times \text{mL}}{15 \text{ gtts} \times \text{min}} = \frac{4 \text{ mL}}{\text{min}} = 4 \text{ mL/min}$$

$$V = R \times T = \frac{4 \text{ mL} \times 15 \text{ min}}{\text{min}} = 60 \text{ mL}$$

4. Note: You must determine the volume (per minute) administered with the 60 gtts/ml set running at 15 gtts. Then determine the gtts (/min) with the 45 gtts/mL set necessary to administer the same volume.

$$R = 15 \text{ gtts/min (60 gtts/mL)} = \frac{15 \text{ gtts} \times \text{mL}}{60 \text{ gtts} \times \text{min}} = \frac{0.25 \text{ mL}}{\text{min}} = 0.25 \text{ mL/min}$$

$$T = 1 \text{ min}$$
$$V = ?$$
$$D = 45 \text{ gtts/mL}$$

$$V = R \times T = \frac{0.25 \text{ mL} \times 1 \text{ min}}{\text{min}} = 0.25 \text{ mL}$$

$$R = \frac{0.25 \text{ mL} \times 45 \text{ gtts}}{\text{min} \times \text{mL}} = \frac{11.25 \text{ gtts}}{\text{min}} = 11.25 \text{ gtts/min}$$

CHAPTER 7: Musculoskeletal Trauma

CONTENT SELF-EVALUATION

MULTIPLE CHOICE

1.	E	p. 211	25.	B	p. 226	49.	C	p. 244
2.	B	p. 212	26.	A	p. 226	50.	D	p. 244
3.	C	p. 212	27.	E	p. 228	51.	B	p. 245
4.	B	p. 212	28.	B	p. 228	52.	B	p. 245
5.	A	p. 212	29.	A	p. 229	53.	E	p. 245
6.	C	p. 213	30.	A	p. 230	54.	E	p. 245
7.	D	p. 213	31.	E	p. 230	55.	D	p. 246
8.	A	p. 214	32.	B	p. 231	56.	E	p. 247
9.	B	p. 214	33.	A	p. 231	57.	D	p. 248
10.	D	p. 214	34.	C	p. 231	58.	E	p. 249
11.	A	p. 215	35.	A	p. 232	59.	B	p. 250
12.	C	p. 217	36.	D	p. 232	60.	A	p. 250
13.	A	p. 217	37.	A	p. 234	61.	B	p. 251
14.	C	p. 217	38.	E	p. 234	62.	C	p. 251
15.	A	p. 218	39.	E	p. 236	63.	C	p. 252
16.	E	p. 218	40.	C	p. 237	64.	A	p. 252
17.	D	p. 218	41.	C	p. 237	65.	A	p. 253
18.	C	p. 219	42.	B	p. 238	66.	B	p. 253
19.	E	p. 219	43.	A	p. 239	67.	E	p. 254
20.	D	p. 223	44.	A	p. 239	68.	E	p. 255
21.	A	p. 224	45.	A	p. 239	69.	D	p. 256
22.	A	p. 225	46.	E	p. 240	70.	B	p. 257
23.	C	p. 225	47.	A	p. 242			
24.	B	p. 225	48.	D	p. 242			

SPECIAL PROJECTS: Recognizing Bones and Bone Injuries

Part I

A. mandible
B. sternum
C. scapula
D. humerus
E. radius
F. ulna
G. sacrum
H. metacarpals
I. tibia
J. fibula

Part II

A. comminuted
B. impacted
C. greenstick
D. oblique
E. spiral
F. transverse

CHAPTER 8: Head, Facial, and Neck Trauma

CONTENT SELF-EVALUATION

MULTIPLE CHOICE

1.	A	p. 263	30.	C	p. 279	59.	B	p. 297
2.	D	p. 263	31.	D	p. 280	60.	E	p. 298
3.	E	p. 264	32.	B	p. 280	61.	A	p. 298
4.	B	p. 264	33.	B	p. 280	62.	C	p. 299
5.	C	p. 265	34.	B	p. 280	63.	B	p. 300
6.	E	p. 266	35.	A	p. 281	64.	E	p. 300
7.	D	p. 266	36.	D	p. 282	65.	B	p. 301
8.	B	p. 267	37.	E	p. 282	66.	B	p. 301
9.	B	p. 267	38.	B	p. 283	67.	D	p. 301
10.	A	p. 268	39.	C	p. 283	68.	E	p. 301
11.	B	p. 268	40.	E	p. 284	69.	A	p. 303
12.	C	p. 268	41.	C	p. 284	70.	B	p. 304
13.	A	p. 268	42.	A	p. 285	71.	A	p. 305
14.	A	p. 268	43.	B	p. 285	72.	A	p. 305
15.	E	p. 269	44.	C	p. 285	73.	E	p. 307
16.	C	p. 269	45.	C	p. 286	74.	B	p. 307
17.	D	p. 270	46.	A	p. 287	75.	A	p. 307
18.	E	p. 270	47.	E	p. 287	76.	D	p. 309
19.	B	p. 271	48.	A	p. 287	77.	B	p. 310
20.	C	p. 273	49.	C	p. 288	78.	C	p. 310
21.	C	p. 273	50.	A	p. 289	79.	B	p. 310
22.	D	p. 274	51.	A	p. 289	80.	D	p. 312
23.	A	p. 274	52.	A	p. 290	81.	B	p. 313
24.	A	p. 274	53.	C	p. 290	82.	B	p. 313
25.	C	p. 274	54.	E	p. 291	83.	E	p. 314
26.	E	p. 275	55.	E	p. 292	84.	C	p. 314
27.	C	p. 278	56.	A	p. 293	85.	B	p. 317
28.	B	p. 278	57.	C	p. 294			
29.	E	p. 278	58.	C	p. 294			

SPECIAL PROJECTS: Crossword Puzzle

Completing a Radio Message and Run Report

Your reports should include most of the following elements.

Radio message from the scene to medical control:

Unit 765 to medical command. We are en route to community hospital with a victim of a one-car auto accident—frontal impact. The patient was reported as initially unconscious but was conscious and alert, though somewhat disoriented upon our arrival. He is now unconscious and responsive only to painful stimuli. He did complain of chest pain that varied with breathing; breath sounds are clear; ECG with NSR at 70. He has a small contusion on his forehead. Vitals are BP 136/88, pulse 52, respirations 22 and deep, and SaO_2 98%. We have established an IV with 1,000 mL NS running TKO and have applied O_2. A cervical collar has been applied and spinal immobilization is underway.

Follow-up radio message to medical control:

Unit 765 to Medical Center. Our patient remains unconscious and responsive only to deep painful stimuli. He is orally intubated with assisted respirations via bag-valve mask @ 25. Current vitals: BP 142/92, pulse 62, and SaO_2 99%. ETA 15 minutes

Ambulance report form:

Please review the next page and ensure that your form includes the appropriate information.

CHAPTER 9: Spinal Trauma

CONTENT SELF-EVALUATION

MULTIPLE CHOICE

1.	B	p. 323	16.	E	p. 335	31.	A	p. 347
2.	C	p. 323	17.	A	p. 336	32.	A	p. 347
3.	B	p. 325	18.	A	p. 337	33.	E	p. 347
4.	B	p. 326	19.	B	p. 337	34.	B	p. 348
5.	A	p. 326	20.	C	p. 337	35.	B	p. 347
6.	C	p. 327	21.	A	p. 338	36.	B	p. 351
7.	A	p. 327	22.	E	p. 339	37.	E	p. 352
8.	E	p. 327	23.	A	p. 339	38.	A	p. 353
9.	B	p. 328	24.	D	p. 340	39.	A	p. 355
10.	C	p. 329	25.	B	p. 341	40.	A	p. 356
11.	A	p. 329	26.	A	p. 342	41.	B	p. 357
12.	A	p. 330	27.	C	p. 342	42.	A	p. 358
13.	E	p. 331	28.	A	p. 343	43.	E	p. 360
14.	D	p. 331	29.	A	p. 345	44.	D	p. 361
15.	A	p. 333	30.	E	p. 345	45.	B	p. 361

SPECIAL PROJECTS:
Recognizing Spinal Regions

A. Cervical, 7
B. Thoracic, 12
C. Lumbar, 5
D. Sacral, 5 (fused into 1)
E. Coccygeal, 5 (fused into 2 or 3)

Dermatome Recognition

C-3   the collar region
T-1   the little finger
T-4   the nipple
T-10   the umbilicus
S-1   the little toe

CHAPTER 10: Thoracic Trauma

CONTENT SELF-EVALUATION

MULTIPLE CHOICE

1.	B	p. 366	26.	C	p. 382	51.	D	p. 395
2.	E	p. 368	27.	D	p. 383	52.	B	p. 395
3.	B	p. 368	28.	B	p. 383	53.	A	p. 395
4.	E	p. 368	29.	A	p. 383	54.	C	p. 396
5.	C	p. 369	30.	A	p. 384	55.	B	p. 396
6.	A	p. 370	31.	E	p. 384	56.	E	p. 396
7.	D	p. 369	32.	B	p. 385	57.	C	p. 396
8.	B	p. 370	33.	D	p. 386	58.	B	p. 397
9.	E	p. 370	34.	B	p. 386	59.	A	p. 397
10.	B	p. 370	35.	B	p. 387	60.	B	p. 398
11.	A	p. 371	36.	E	p. 386	61.	E	p. 398
12.	B	p. 372	37.	D	p. 389	62.	E	p. 399
13.	C	p. 372	38.	B	p. 389	63.	A	p. 400
14.	C	p. 372	39.	D	p. 389	64.	D	p. 401
15.	E	p. 372	40.	C	p. 390	65.	E	p. 402
16.	E	p. 374	41.	D	p. 391	66.	B	p. 402
17.	B	p. 375	42.	E	p. 391	67.	B	p. 403
18.	B	p. 375	43.	C	p. 391	68.	A	p. 405
19.	C	p. 376	44.	A	p. 392	69.	D	p. 405
20.	A	p. 377	45.	A	p. 392	70.	B	p. 406
21.	C	p. 378	46.	A	p. 393	71.	B	p. 406
22.	D	p. 379	47.	D	p. 394	72.	C	p. 406
23.	B	p. 379	48.	A	p. 394	73.	A	p. 408
24.	D	p. 379	49.	E	p. 395	74.	B	p. 409
25.	A	p. 380	50.	B	p. 395	75.	E	p. 410

SPECIAL PROJECTS: Labeling Diagrams

Part I

A. sternum
B. lung
C. heart
D. trachea
E. pleura
F. ribs
G. diaphragm
H. pleural space

Part II

1.	A	5.	G	9.	F
2.	H	6.	E	10.	C
3.	K	7.	B	11.	I
4.	D	8.	J		

Problem Solving—Chest Injury

Signs and symptoms of tension pneumothorax: mechanism of injury, progressive dyspnea, diminished breath sounds on injured side, JVD, tracheal deviation away from injury, subcutaneous emphysema, hyperresonant percussion on injured side, signs and symptoms of shock.

Patient report should include: chest trauma patient, unequal breath sounds, side involved, progressive dyspnea, JVD.

Decompression attempt location: between 2nd and 3rd ribs (2nd intercostal space) midclavicular line of side with decreased breath sounds.

Date Today's Date	Emergency Medical Services Run Report	Run # 913

Patient Information / Service Information / Times

Patient Information	Service Information	Times
Name: John	Agency: Unit 765	Rcvd 02:15
Address:	Location: Hwy 127 & Cty Tr H	Enrt 02:15
City: St: Zip:	Call Origin: 911 Center	Scne 02:32
Age: 31 Birth: / / Sex: [M][F]	Type: Emrg[X] Non[ ] Trnsfr[ ]	LvSn 02:42
Nature of Call: One-car auto accident/frontal impact		ArHsp 03:15
Chief Complaint: Chest pain which varies with resp./unconsciousness		InSv 03:35

Description of Current Problem:

Pt. is a 31 y.o. male victim of an auto accident. He impacted the steering wheel and windshield. Though initially unconscious, the pt. was conscious, alert, though disoriented upon our arrival, and complaining of chest pain only. During extrication his left pupil dilated, his level of consciousness began to drop, and he became unresponsive. Physical assessment did reveal a small contusion on his forehead with limited swelling and no crepitation.

Medical Problems

Past		Present
[ ]	Cardiac	[ ]
[ ]	Stroke	[ ]
[ ]	Acute Abdomen	[ ]
[ ]	Diabetes	[ ]
[ ]	Psychiatric	[ ]
[ ]	Epilepsy	[ ]
[ ]	Drug/Alcohol	[ ]
[ ]	Poisoning	[ ]
[ ]	Allergy/Asthma	[ ]
[ ]	Syncope	[ ]
[ ]	Obstetrical	[ ]
[ ]	GYN	[ ]

Other: none

Trauma Scr: 12   Glasgow: 14/5

On Scene Care:	First Aid: None
C-collar, spinal imm.	
Oxygen, IV 16 ga L forearm – NS	Police report the patient was unconscious
8.0 mm ET tube digital, assisted resp @	when they arrived.
16 via BVM @ 15 L O$_2$	By Whom?

O2 @ 10 L 02:36 Via NRB	C-Collar 02:34	S-Immob. 02:33	Stretcher 02:42

Allergies/Meds: None	Past Med Hx: None

Time	Pulse	Resp.	BP S/D	LOC	ECG
02:36	R: 70 [X][i]	R: 20 [s][l]	124/88	[X][v][p][u]	NSR SaO$_2$ 99%

Care/Comments: Conscious and alert, chest pain on resp, clear breath sounds 16 ga IV/NS

02:41	R: 52 [X][i]	R: 22 [s][X]	136/88	[a][v][p][u]	NSR SaO$_2$ 98%

Care/Comments: Pt. becomes unconscious, responds to painful stimuli, left pupil is dilated

02:51	R: 62 [X][i]	R: 24 [s][X]	142/92	[a][v][p][u]	NSR SaO$_2$ 97% GCS 5

Care/Comments: Pt. is unconscious, 8.0 ET tube – BVM hyperventilating

03:01	R: 50 [X][i]	R: 25 [s][X]	140/90	[a][v][p][u]	NSR SaO$_2$ 97%

Care/Comments: Pt. is unresponsive to all but painful stimuli

Destination: Medical Center	Personnel:	Certification
Reason:[ ]pt [ ]Closest [X]M.D. [ ]Other	1. Jan	[R][E][O]
Contacted: [X]Radio [ ]Tele [ ]Direct	2. Steve	[R][E][O]
Ar Status: [X]Better [ ]UnC [X]Worse	3.	[P][R][O]

CHAPTER 11: Abdominal Trauma

CONTENT SELF-EVALUATION

MULTIPLE CHOICE

1. A *p. 416*	18. A *p. 425*	35. A *p. 432*
2. C *p. 416*	19. B *p. 425*	36. A *p. 432*
3. E *p. 416*	20. B *p. 426*	37. E *p. 432*
4. E *p. 416*	21. D *p. 426*	38. D *p. 432*
5. B *p. 416*	22. C *p. 426*	39. D *p. 432*
6. A *p. 418*	23. B *p. 427*	40. C *p. 433*
7. E *p. 416*	24. E *p. 427*	41. B *p. 436*
8. A *p. 419*	25. C *p. 427*	42. C *p. 436*
9. C *p. 418*	26. A *p. 428*	43. D *p. 436*
10. B *p. 419*	27. C *p. 428*	44. C *p. 439*
11. B *p. 420*	28. B *p. 428*	45. C *p. 440*
12. D *p. 420*	29. A *p. 429*	46. D *p. 440*
13. C *p. 422*	30. D *p. 429*	47. B *p. 440*
14. D *p. 422*	31. E *p. 430*	48. D *p. 440*
15. C *p. 423*	32. E *p. 430*	49. A *p. 442*
16. C *p. 424*	33. D *p. 431*	50. A *p. 442*
17. D *p. 424*	34. C *p. 431*	

SPECIAL PROJECT: Writing a Run Report

Please review the next page and ensure that your form includes the appropriate information.

CHAPTER 12: Shock Trauma Resuscitation

CONTENT SELF-EVALUATION

MULTIPLE CHOICE

1. D *p. 446*	21. A *p. 457*	41. D *p. 469*
2. E *p. 447*	22. C *p. 457*	42. A *p. 470*
3. E *p. 449*	23. A *p. 458*	43. D *p. 472*
4. B *p. 449*	24. C *p. 458*	44. D *p. 471*
5. E *p. 450*	25. B *p. 458*	45. D *p. 471*
6. D *p. 450*	26. B *p. 459*	46. A *p. 475*
7. A *p. 451*	27. E *p. 459*	47. B *p. 475*
8. D *p. 452*	28. A *p. 459*	48. B *p. 476*
9. B *p. 453*	29. E *p. 460*	49. C *p. 476*
10. B *p. 453*	30. E *p. 461*	50. A *p. 477*
11. B *p. 453*	31. A *p. 462*	51. A *p. 478*
12. E *p. 454*	32. B *p. 462*	52. E *p. 478*
13. D *p. 455*	33. D *p. 463*	53. A *p. 479*
14. A *p. 455*	34. E *p. 464*	54. B *p. 480*
15. E *p. 455*	35. A *p. 465*	55. A *p. 481*
16. E *p. 455*	36. C *p. 466*	56. B *p. 482*
17. A *p. 456*	37. D *p. 467*	57. D *p. 483*
18. D *p. 456*	38. B *p. 468*	58. B *p. 483*
19. B *p. 457*	39. A *p. 469*	59. B *p. 484*
20. B *p. 457*	40. C *p. 469*	60. E *p. 486*

SPECIAL PROJECT: Crossword Puzzle

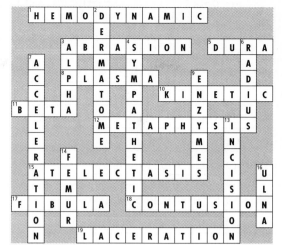

TRAUMA EMERGENCIES: Content Review

CONTENT SELF-EVALUATION

CHAPTER 1: Trauma and Trauma Systems

1. B *p. 5*	5. C *p. 9*	9. A *p. 11*
2. B *p. 5*	6. D *p. 10*	10. E *p. 12*
3. B *p. 6*	7. A *p. 10*	
4. A *p. 7*	8. B *p. 11*	

CHAPTER 2: Blunt Trauma

11. A *p. 20*	18. C *p. 29*	25. B *p. 45*
12. B *p. 22*	19. B *p. 32*	26. E *p. 46*
13. C *p. 23*	20. C *p. 35*	27. A *p. 47*
14. D *p. 24*	21. A *p. 37*	28. A *p. 49*
15. E *p. 26*	22. C *p. 39*	29. A *p. 49*
16. B *p. 26*	23. A *p. 40*	30. E *p. 51*
17. E *p. 27*	24. A *p. 45*	

CHAPTER 3: Penetrating Trauma

31. A *p. 57*	36. D *p. 66*	41. E *p. 70*
32. B *p. 57*	37. A *p. 67*	42. A *p. 71*
33. A *p. 59*	38. E *p. 67*	43. C *p. 71*
34. C *p. 62*	39. A *p. 69*	44. A *p. 71*
35. B *p. 64*	40. A *p. 70*	45. B *p. 74*

CHAPTER 4: Hemorrhage and Shock

46. B *p. 79*	56. D *p. 90*	66. B *p. 106*
47. E *p. 79*	57. C *p. 91*	67. C *p. 108*
48. B *p. 81*	58. A *p. 93*	68. A *p. 108*
49. A *p. 81*	59. A *p. 94*	69. D *p. 109*
50. A *p. 81*	60. D *p. 95*	70. B *p. 110*
51. A *p. 82*	61. B *p. 96*	71. C *p. 111*
52. B *p. 83*	62. E *p. 101*	72. A *p. 112*
53. B *p. 84*	63. B *p. 102*	73. A *p. 113*
54. E *p. 85*	64. E *p. 104*	74. C *p. 116*
55. B *p. 88*	65. C *p. 105*	75. C *p. 116*

Date Today's Date	Emergency Medical Services Run Report	Run # 914

Patient Information

Name: Marty		
Address: Harborview Apts #112		
City:	St:	Zip:
Age: 43 Birth: / /	Sex: [M] [F]	

Nature of Call: Shots fired

Chief Complaint: "Shot by wife"

Service Information / Times

Agency:	Rcvd	03:25
Location: Harborview Apts #112	Enrt	03:25
Call Origin: 911 Center	Scne	03:32
Type: Emrg [X] Non [ ] Trnsfr [ ]	LvSn	03:38
	ArHsp	03:47
	InSv	04:00

Description of Current Problem:

Shot by a 9mm handgun @ close range.

Wound to LUQ, oozing small amount of blood.

No apparent exit wound(s). Describes pain as sharp.

Surrounding area feels "burning" in nature.

Medical Problems

Past		Present
[ ]	Cardiac	[ ]
[ ]	Stroke	[ ]
[ ]	Acute Abdomen	[ ]
[ ]	Diabetes	[ ]
[ ]	Psychiatric	[ ]
[X]	Epilepsy	[ ]
[ ]	Drug/Alcohol	[ ]
[ ]	Poisoning	[ ]
[ ]	Allergy/Asthma	[ ]
[ ]	Syncope	[ ]
[ ]	Obstetrical	[ ]
[ ]	GYN	[ ]

Other:

Trauma Scr: 12   Glasgow: 15

On Scene Care: Covered wound w/ sterile dressing, moved to stretcher – IV 14 ga angio (L) antecubital w/ 1,000 LR	First Aid: Towel – patient seated against wall
	By Whom? unknown

02 @ 12 L 03:35 Via NRM	C-Collar N/A	S-Immob. N/A	Stretcher 03:36

Allergies/Meds: Phenobarbital Dilantin no allergies, Tetanus – 3 yrs ago	Past Med Hx: Seizures – controlled

Time	Pulse	Resp.	BP S/D	LOC	ECG
03:35	R: 80 [X][i]	R: 22 [s][l]	110/86	[X][v][p][u]	NSR SaO2 99%

Care/Comments: A/O x 3   O2 12 L/NRM   IV 1,000 LR

03:42	R: 86 [X][i]	R: 24 [X][l]	112/86	[X][v][p][u]	NSR SaO2 99%

Care/Comments: Shoulder pain & thirst; BJ: clear in all fields; no bowel sounds

03:47	R: 88 [r][i]	R: 22 [X][l]	112/92	[X][v][p][u]	

Care/Comments: Pt. transport uneventful

:	R: [r][i]	R: [s][l]	/	[a][v][p][u]	

Care/Comments:

Destination: St. Joseph's Hospital	Personnel:	Certification
Reason: [ ]pt [ ]Closest [X]M.D. [ ]Other	1. Janice	[R][E][O]
Contacted: [X]Radio [ ]Tele [ ]Direct	2. Doug	[R][E][O]
Ar Status: [ ]Better [X]UnC [ ]Worse	3.	[P][E][O]

CHAPTER 5: Soft-Tissue Trauma

76.	B	p. 127	88.	B	p. 139	100.	E	p. 154
77.	C	p. 126	89.	B	p. 139	101.	E	p. 155
78.	D	p. 128	90.	C	p. 140	102.	D	p. 156
79.	C	p. 129	91.	E	p. 141	103.	A	p. 157
80.	A	p. 129	92.	D	p. 142	104.	B	p. 158
81.	A	p. 130	93.	E	p. 142	105.	D	p. 160
82.	D	p. 132	94.	B	p. 143	106.	C	p. 161
83.	E	p. 133	95.	B	p. 144	107.	A	p. 163
84.	E	p. 133	96.	A	p. 145	108.	B	p. 164
85.	E	p. 135	97.	A	p. 147	109.	A	p. 165
86.	C	p. 138	98.	A	p. 147	110.	E	p. 168
87.	A	p. 138	99.	B	p. 148			

CHAPTER 6: Burns

111.	B	p. 172	123.	A	p. 185	135.	B	p. 196
112.	A	p. 173	124.	C	p. 186	136.	B	p. 196
113.	D	p. 175	125.	B	p. 186	137.	B	p. 197
114.	A	p. 176	126.	C	p. 186	138.	B	p. 197
115.	C	p. 176	127.	E	p. 186	139.	D	p. 198
116.	A	p. 178	128.	B	p. 192	140.	D	p. 199
117.	A	p. 179	129.	A	p. 192	141.	B	p. 199
118.	B	p. 180	130.	E	p. 193	142.	E	p. 200
119.	B	p. 180	131.	B	p. 195	143.	C	p. 202
120.	A	p. 183	132.	B	p. 195	144.	B	p. 203
121.	C	p. 183	133.	D	p. 195	145.	C	p. 204
122.	B	p. 183	134.	C	p. 195			

CHAPTER 7: Musculoskeletal Trauma

146.	E	p. 211	161.	E	p. 226	176.	B	p. 245
147.	A	p. 212	162.	E	p. 229	177.	E	p. 245
148.	B	p. 213	163.	A	p. 230	178.	A	p. 245
149.	E	p. 212	164.	C	p. 230	179.	B	p. 246
150.	C	p. 212	165.	B	p. 232	180.	B	p. 247
151.	E	p. 214	166.	C	p. 232	181.	E	p. 249
152.	C	p. 215	167.	B	p. 234	182.	C	p. 250
153.	B	p. 218	168.	E	p. 235	183.	B	p. 252
154.	C	p. 218	169.	C	p. 237	184.	D	p. 253
155.	B	p. 218	170.	B	p. 238	185.	E	p. 253
156.	C	p. 219	171.	A	p. 239	186.	A	p. 253
157.	E	p. 222	172.	B	p. 239	187.	E	p. 254
158.	B	p. 223	173.	B	p. 242	188.	E	p. 255
159.	C	p. 223	174.	D	p. 242	189.	E	p. 256
160.	C	p. 225	175.	B	p. 244	190.	B	p. 257

CHAPTER 8: Head, Facial, and Neck Trauma

191.	A	p. 263	210.	A	p. 280	229.	D	p. 301
192.	A	p. 264	211.	A	p. 282	230.	B	p. 301
193.	B	p. 266	212.	E	p. 282	231.	B	p. 301
194.	A	p. 266	213.	B	p. 283	232.	A	p. 303
195.	E	p. 267	214.	A	p. 284	233.	A	p. 304
196.	B	p. 266	215.	A	p. 285	234.	A	p. 304
197.	C	p. 268	216.	A	p. 285	235.	A	p. 304
198.	A	p. 268	217.	C	p. 285	236.	D	p. 305
199.	A	p. 268	218.	B	p. 286	237.	E	p. 307
200.	B	p. 270	219.	D	p. 287	238.	A	p. 307
201.	A	p. 270	220.	A	p. 288	239.	A	p. 309
202.	A	p. 271	221.	B	p. 289	240.	C	p. 310
203.	E	p. 272	222.	C	p. 290	241.	A	p. 310
204.	B	p. 273	223.	E	p. 292	242.	D	p. 312
205.	E	p. 274	224.	E	p. 293	243.	A	p. 313
206.	B	p. 274	225.	B	p. 294	244.	C	p. 314
207.	B	p. 275	226.	B	p. 297	245.	A	p. 315
208.	A	p. 278	227.	B	p. 298			
209.	B	p. 279	228.	A	p. 300			

CHAPTER 9: Spinal Trauma

246.	A	p. 325	256.	A	p. 336	266.	D	p. 343
247.	A	p. 325	257.	A	p. 337	267.	D	p. 345
248.	C	p. 327	258.	A	p. 337	268.	C	p. 347
249.	B	p. 326	259.	B	p. 338	269.	C	p. 347
250.	D	p. 329	260.	E	p. 339	270.	E	p. 362
251.	B	p. 329	261.	E	p. 339	271.	A	p. 352
252.	B	p. 331	262.	E	p. 340	272.	A	p. 353
253.	C	p. 331	263.	A	p. 341	273.	B	p. 354
254.	D	p. 335	264.	B	p. 342	274.	C	p. 358
255.	B	p. 333	265.	C	p. 342	275.	B	p. 358

CHAPTER 10: Thoracic Trauma

276.	B	p. 366	290.	C	p. 382	304.	E	p. 396
277.	E	p. 368	291.	D	p. 382	305.	D	p. 396
278.	C	p. 370	292.	D	p. 383	306.	A	p. 397
279.	A	p. 370	293.	D	p. 384	307.	D	p. 397
280.	B	p. 370	294.	A	p. 386	308.	C	p. 398
281.	C	p. 372	295.	A	p. 386	309.	D	p. 398
282.	E	p. 372	296.	A	p. 389	310.	A	p. 400
283.	D	p. 372	297.	A	p. 390	311.	C	p. 402
284.	A	p. 372	298.	E	p. 392	312.	A	p. 405
285.	E	p. 375	299.	C	p. 392	313.	B	p. 407
286.	A	p. 377	300.	D	p. 393	314.	A	p. 408
287.	C	p. 378	301.	B	p. 394	315.	B	p. 410
288.	E	p. 379	302.	E	p. 395			
289.	C	p. 379	303.	A	p. 395			

CHAPTER 11: Abdominal Trauma

316.	D	p. 416	325.	B	p. 424	334.	A	p. 430
317.	B	p. 416	326.	E	p. 425	335.	B	p. 432
318.	E	p. 416	327.	A	p. 426	336.	B	p. 432
319.	D	p. 418	328.	B	p. 426	337.	A	p. 433
320.	B	p. 418	329.	B	p. 426	338.	A	p. 436
321.	A	p. 419	330.	C	p. 427	339.	E	p. 437
322.	B	p. 420	331.	B	p. 429	340.	D	p. 440
323.	C	p. 420	332.	B	p. 429			
324.	D	p. 422	333.	B	p. 430			

CHAPTER 12: Shock Trauma Resuscitation

341.	D	p. 446	353.	C	p. 458	365.	B	p. 469
342.	D	p. 446	354.	B	p. 459	366.	A	p. 470
343.	E	p. 449	355.	E	p. 459	367.	B	p. 474
344.	B	p. 452	356.	A	p. 460	368.	D	p. 475
345.	B	p. 453	357.	E	p. 461	369.	B	p. 475
346.	A	p. 453	358.	B	p. 462	370.	D	p. 476
347.	E	p. 454	359.	D	p. 462	371.	D	p. 478
348.	A	p. 455	360.	E	p. 465	372.	D	p. 480
349.	C	p. 455	361.	D	p. 465	373.	E	p. 483
350.	C	p. 457	362.	C	p. 467	374.	D	p. 484
351.	D	p. 457	363.	A	p. 468	375.	E	p. 486
352.	D	p. 457	364.	C	p. 469			

PATIENT SCENARIO FLASHCARDS

The following pages contain prepared 3" × 5" index cards. Each card presents a patient scenario with the appropriate signs and symptoms. On the reverse side are the appropriate field diagnosis and the care steps you should consider providing for your patient.

Detach the pages and cut out the cards and review each of them in detail. If there are any discrepancies with what you have been taught in class, please review these with your instructor and medical director and employ what is appropriate for your EMS system. Record any changes directly on the cards.

Once your cards are prepared and you have reviewed them carefully, shuffle them and then read the scenario and signs and symptoms. Try to identify the patient's problem and the treatment you would employ. Compare your diagnosis and care steps with those on the reverse side of your flashcard. This exercise will help you recognize and remember the common serious trauma emergencies, their presentation, and the appropriate care.

SCENARIO 1:   Your patient is a 36-year-old driver of a small auto that collided with a tree. He was wearing his seat belt, firmly impacted the steering column, and now is complaining of increasing dyspnea.

   S/S: Anxiety
Apprehension
Lowering level of consciousness
Shallow rapid breaths
Pallor
Left breath sounds diminished
Trachea shifted to the right
Hyperresonant percussion right side of chest
Some subcutaneous emphysema in lower neck
Jugular vein distension

SCENARIO 2:   A 47-year-old male driver was injured in a moderate-speed crash. Lateral impact was on the driver's side of the auto.

   S/S: Anxiety
Pulse deficit, left arm
Central chest pain "tearing"
Minor pain, left thorax
Contusions, left thorax
Capillary refill—2 seconds
Clear heart sounds
Pallor
Bilaterally equal breath sounds

SCENARIO 1:

Field Diagnosis: Tension pneumothorax

Management: Scene Size-up—mechanism of injury/index of suspicion
 BSI—gloves
Initial Assessment
 Spinal precautions—Spinal immobilization indicated.
 Calm and reassure patient.
 Airway—Maintain a patent airway.
 Breathing—Provide high-flow oxygen.
 Circulation—Initiate an IV w/ large-bore catheters. Monitor
  ECG. Maintain body temperature. Control obvious
  hemorrhage.
Rapid Trauma Assessment
 Provide pleural decompression with one-way valve. Reassess
  breath sounds and breathing.
Rapid extrication from the vehicle.
Provide ongoing assessment(s).
Provide rapid transport. Alert trauma center.

SCENARIO 2:

Field Diagnosis: Dissecting aortic aneurysm

Management: Scene Size-up—mechanism of injury/index of suspicion
 BSI—gloves
Initial Assessment
 Spinal precautions—Spinal immobilization indicated.
 Calm and reassure patient.
 Airway—Maintain a patent airway.
 Breathing—Provide high-flow oxygen. Consider IPPV.
 Circulation—Initiate an IV w/ large-bore catheters. Administer
  fluids conservatively. Monitor ECG. Maintain body
  temperature.
Rapid Trauma Assessment
 If patient deteriorates, run fluids rapidly.
Rapid extrication from the vehicle.
Provide ongoing assessment(s).
Provide rapid transport. Alert trauma center.

SCENARIO 3:

A young male was involved in a frontal impact auto accident in which he struck the windshield. He is found conscious and alert and seated in the auto but cannot move his legs or arms.

S/S:
Anxiety
Apprehension
Diaphragmatic breathing
Bilateral anesthesia and paralysis
Cool limbs
Blood pressure 96/76
Priapism
Arms move to hold-up position
Capillary refill—2 seconds

SCENARIO 4:

A 34-year-old pedestrian was struck by an auto and thrown to the roadside. She is found complaining of bilateral hip pain and is unable to move her legs.

S/S:
Diaphoresis
Anxiety
Apprehension
Slight dyspnea
Pallor
Pelvic pain
Rapid weak pulse
Pelvic instability
Crepitation with pressure on iliac crests
Capillary refill—4 seconds

SCENARIO 5:

Your patient was involved in a serious frontal impact auto collision with deformity of the steering wheel, though the windshield did not shatter. He is a well-developed male in his mid-thirties.

S/S:
Conscious, alert, and fully oriented.
Crushing substernal chest pain
Anxiety
Strong but irregular pulse
Bilaterally equal breath sounds
Clear heart sounds
ECG—sinus rhythm with frequent PACs
Jugular veins—normal
No tracheal deviation

SCENARIO 3:

Field Diagnosis: Spinal cord injury (midcervical)

Management: Scene Size-up—mechanism of injury/index of suspicion
    BSI—gloves
Initial Assessment
    Spinal precautions—Spinal immobilization indicated.
    Calm and reassure patient.
    Airway—Maintain a patent airway.
    Breathing—Provide high-flow oxygen. Consider IPPV.
    Circulation—Initiate 1 or 2 IVs w/ large-bore catheters.
        Monitor ECG. Maintain body temperature. Control obvious
        hemorrhage.
Rapid Trauma Assessment
    Consider methylprednisolone (30 mg/kg). Consider a fluid
        challenge.
Rapid extrication from the vehicle.
Provide ongoing assessment(s).
Provide gentle transport. Alert trauma center.

SCENARIO 4:

Field Diagnosis: Pelvic fracture

Management: Scene Size-up—mechanism of injury/index of suspicion
    BSI—gloves
Initial Assessment
    Spinal precautions—Spinal immobilization indicated.
    Calm and reassure patient.
    Airway—Maintain a patent airway.
    Breathing—Provide high-flow oxygen.
    Circulation—Initiate 1 or 2 IVs w/ large-bore catheters.
        Monitor ECG. Maintain body temperature. Control
        obvious hemorrhage.
Rapid Trauma Assessment
    Inflate PASG to stabilize pelvis.
Provide ongoing assessment(s).
Provide rapid transport. Alert trauma center.

SCENARIO 5:

Field Diagnosis: Myocardial contusion

Management: Scene Size-up—mechanism of injury/index of suspicion
    BSI—gloves
Initial Assessment
    Spinal precautions—Spinal immobilization indicated.
    Calm and reassure patient.
    Airway—Maintain patent airway.
    Breathing—Provide high-flow oxygen.
    Circulation—Initiate an IV w/ large-bore catheter. Monitor
        ECG. Maintain body temperature. Control any obvious
        hemorrhage.
Rapid Trauma Assessment
    Treat dysrhythmias as per protocol.
Provide ongoing assessment(s).
Provide rapid transport. Alert trauma center.